Exploring your
Anger

FRIEND OR FOE?

Glenn Taylor and Rod Wilson

REGENT COLLEGE PUBLISHING • VANCOUVER

Exploring Your Anger
Copyright © 1997 by Glenn Taylor and Rod Wilson

First published by 1997 by Baker Book House, Grand Rapids, Michigan.

This edition published 2003 by Regent College Publishing
5800 University Boulevard, Vancouver, BC V6T 2E4 Canada
www.regentpublishing.com

All rights reserved. No part of this book may be reproduced in any form without permission in writing from the publisher, except by a reviewer who may quote brief passages in a review to be printed in a magazine or newspaper.

Views expressed in works published by Regent College Publishing are those of the author and do not necessarily represent the views or opinions of Regent College. For more information about Regent College, visit our website: http://www.regent-college.edu

A cataloguing record for this publication is available from the National Library of Canada

ISBN 1-57383-249-9

To our wives, Bev Wilson and Mary Taylor, who along with our children have provided a context of support and acceptance for exploring human relationships including the understanding and expression of anger.

Other books in the Strategic Christian Living series

Douglas McMurry and Everett L. Worthington, Jr., *Value Your Mate: How to Strengthen Your Marriage*

Daniel R. Green and Mel Lawrenz, *Why Do I Feel Like Hiding? How to Overcome Shame and Guilt*

James R. Beck and David T. Moore, *Why Worry? Conquering a Common Inclination*

Harold Wahking and Gene Zimmerman, *Fulfilled Sexuality: How to Find Help and Hope for Difficulties*

Siang-Yang Tan and John Ortberg, Jr., *Coping with Depression: The Common Cold of the Emotional Life*

Gary Steven Shogren and Edward T. Welch, *Running in Circles: How to Find Freedom from Addictive Behavior*

Mel Lawrenz and Daniel Green, *Life after Grief: How to Survive Loss and Trauma*

Everett L. Worthington, Jr., and Kirby Worthington, *Value Your Children: Becoming Better Parental Disciplemakers*

David Benner and Robert Harvey, *Choosing the Gift of Forgiveness: How to Overcome Hurts and Brokenness*

CONTENTS

1. Christians and Anger: Friends or Foes?   7
2. Charting a Course: Exploring Your Anger   31
3. The Power of Feelings: Sin or Righteousness?   53
4. Triggers and Thoughts: Thinking Effectively About Your Anger   73
5. Avoiding Vengeance: Behaving Righteously   95

   Endnotes   109
   References   110
   For Further Reading   111

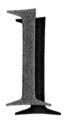

CHRISTIANS AND ANGER
FRIENDS OR FOES?

> Summary: The saints at Mountainview Bible Church are similar to Christians in most churches. They all struggle with anger, but each person experiences and expresses it differently. As a church they purport to live by biblical standards so it is important that they understand the teaching about anger in the Scriptures. Then they can determine whether anger is a friend or foe.

A Day in the Life of Mountainview Bible Church

It was a typical Sunday in the life of Mountainview Bible Church. The worship was expressive, the sermon riveting, and the interaction substantial. But there was more going on than meets the eye. William was sitting in the back pew and he was frustrated. His beloved Buffalo Bills had just lost the Super Bowl last Sunday and he was reviewing video replays in his head and bemoaning another loss. Then there was Sally. Sitting in the middle of the section by the window, she was steamed. The woman directly in front of her was raising her hands in worship during the singing and Sally was beside herself. Why would anyone want to bring this much attention to themselves and disrupt everyone around them?! On the other side of the sanctuary sat Judith. A single mom, she had spent most of the morning screaming at her children and she was in recovery. The irritation had subsided to some degree, but her heart was still racing and she was conscious of those dreaded red lines running up her neck. Up on the platform sat Helmut, the soloist for the morning. As he looked out over the congregation he spotted Bonnie, the woman who had refused his many invitations for a date. As he prepared to sing a moving song by Twila Paris, he was very aware of his anger toward Bonnie and her stubborn attitude. And then there was Elisabeth. When Doreen got up to give the announcement about the women's retreat she could feel exasperation welling up inside. Why does she have to talk like that in public and draw so much attention to herself?! And, of course, in his usual seat, second from the front, sat Tom. His major task during worship was to count the number of hymns and choruses and decide whether the former was being sacrificed for the sake of the latter. In this particular service, he was provoked because the ratio did not fit his tried and true personal preferences.

It really was a typical day in the life of Mountainview Bible Church. But William's frustration, Sally's steam, Judith's irritation, Helmut's anger, Elisabeth's exasperation, and Tom's provocation probably describe a typical day in the life of most churches on most Sundays. While melodious words are sung and powerful sermons are spoken, anger is often not far below the surface. In fact, it is often very much at the surface.

At the back of the church after the service, William and Sally greet each other and share a few pleasantries. Eventually Sally blurts out, "Could you believe that woman with her hands in the air during the singing this morning? Doesn't that kind of thing really get to you?" William, who had been oblivious to the obvious during the service, provides a rather unhelpful response, "I didn't see her." "You didn't see her? How could you miss that obvious display of self-centeredness?" Sally storms off with another incident to add to her anger bag and William is left with a vague feeling that he did not give her what she wanted. Then he has the unfortunate experience of running into Tom.

"What did you think of the service today, William?" asks Tom, hoping that his friend will bring the same criteria to bear that he considers to be important. "Not bad, I guess," answers William. "Not bad? Aren't you getting a little tired of all the choruses we are singing? I get the impression that the overhead is now a requirement if we are going to worship." At that point Tom catches the eye of someone else and moves over to talk to them. William decides it is probably time for him to move toward the parking lot. On his way he passes Helmut and Elisabeth, both of whom are friendly and greet him warmly.

Anger as a Personal and Individual Experience

You have to feel sorry for William, who had been using the morning service to meditate on fumbles, interceptions, and missed field goals. How was he going to make judgments on worship styles or music preferences? However, on the way home he did some reflecting. Neither of these things makes him angry. He likes it when people express themselves physically in worship. They seem more into it, more responsive, more moved. So many people seem overly dull and reflective in worship. He wishes more people would raise their hands. He understands the chorus/hymn problem, but it is not an emotional subject for him. He likes the blend of the contemporary and the traditional. But if you want to talk about a running play on third down with four to go, that is a different story!

What does this scenario tell us about anger? Anger is personal and individual. William did not share Sally's anger about raised hands or Tom's frustration with the number of choruses. Obviously, Helmut's personal experience with Bonnie could not be shared by William since he was not being rejected. By the same token, Judith's exasperation with her children was unique to her and since William did not have children he could not fully understand it.

What makes anger personal? We will answer that in more detail in the next chapter but let us start by trying to understand the dynamics of anger through a simple working definition:

> Anger is an experience that occurs when a goal, value, or expectation that I have chosen has been blocked or when my sense of personal worth is threatened.

First of all, we need to understand that anger is a feeling, an emotional experience. When we say things like, "She makes my blood boil" or "He gets under my skin," we are describing physiological reactions and deep feelings. Feelings are personal and unique for each of us. One of us might watch a football game and experience great frustration when our team loses. Another person might watch the same game and feel great elation because they were pulling for the opposing team. A third person may find football boring and never turn on the game. Three unique feelings—frustration, elation, and boredom—are all in response to the same event.

We need to realize that anger is tied to our goals, values, or expectations that are resident in our thinking. Where do these come from? They find their roots in our personal heritage and history. One person has learned to value particular styles of expression in worship. Another has learned to be committed to variety in worship and is never frustrated with anyone in the service as long as they are worshiping. A third has always perceived the worship time as the appetizer before the main meal sermon. For them, little value is accorded to the early part of the service. With unique goals, values, and expectations, these three individuals will come to the same event with a personal perspective.

Anger is not just confined to feelings and thinking. It also is connected to our will. We are not the victims of our goals, values, and expectations. As a result of our historical experience, we have learned to choose and cherish particular viewpoints. A mother has grown up to believe that respect and obedience to parents is an important value. She has decided to own that and it has become incorporated into her approach to life. In the presence of children who are insolent and unruly, this mother will experience frustration. Her feeling can be traced to the discrepancy between her goals and values and the behavior of her children. In contrast, a mother who has not chosen to make respect and obedience a high value may find insolence inconvenient, but it will not produce anger.

Because feelings, thinking, and will vary from person to person, we can expect that the experience of anger will be personal and individual. It would be impossible for everyone to experience anger in the same way at the same circumstance.

Anger as a Personal and Individual Expression

It is important to draw a distinction between the experience of anger and the expression of anger. Various individuals at Mountainview Bible Church were experiencing anger, albeit in unique ways. However, their expression of the anger varied. William never told anyone about his frustration at the Bills' loss, Judith kept her irritation to herself, Sally and Tom used William as a dumping ground for their anger after the service. Elisabeth and Helmut are friendly to William and do not communicate their exasperation. As is the case with the experience of anger, the expression of it is as varied as the individuals acting on it. At least four major expressions are possible:

1. Suppression
2. Repression
3. Expression
4. Confession

The suppression of anger is a process that takes the experience of anger seriously but holds down its expression. Take the case of Elisabeth. She is angry with Doreen when Doreen is giving a public announcement in the service. It is probably appropriate for her to suppress the expression of anger and not disrupt the service by standing up and letting her have it. However, for her to continue to suppress the anger and never deal with it is probably not helpful for either of them. Suppression then is an appropriate way to handle anger if the situation warrants it.

The repression of anger occurs when people ignore and deny their experience to such a degree that they are unable to express it behaviorally or even acknowledge it to themselves. Others may even sense that the individual is angry and frustrated, but the person is very much out of touch with what is happening. This approach to the expression of anger is never appropriate. To block and deny what one is experiencing is to live a lie.

Both Tom and Sally expressed their anger to William at the back of the church. They revealed their emotions in direct ways and exposed some of the values and expectations that were lurking behind the feelings. In contrast to suppression and repression where there is a separation between experience and expression, expression is a form of anger management that does not draw this distinction. However, whether this is always an appropriate way to deal with anger is a point that could be debated.

Imagine Tom phoning William after the service and in a calm manner describing the irritation he was experiencing in the service. In this scenario, Tom would be confessing his anger. He would not be letting all the emotions out, but would simply be talking about his experience in a somewhat detached manner. Often the confession of anger involves an exposure of the blocked values and goals without any of the richness of feeling that comes with that violation.

How Should Christians Respond?

Mountainview Bible Church, as its name implies, seeks to extol the virtues of a righteous life that is in harmony with Scripture. So how do they deal with the Toms and the Sallys, the Helmuts and the Williams? Some in the church have adopted the "personality orientation." They see anger as a function of personality, without having much significance: "She's like that, you know. I have known her family for years. It's just the way they react." Others have adopted the "tolerance orientation." Anger is something to be tolerated in others, and any struggle with others' anger is interpreted to reflect a lack of patience and understanding. Some have bought into the "contagious orientation." In the presence of anger they will gather around and begin to fan the flame by joining in with the critique and assessment. The "denial orientation" is strong for some in the church. Even when others are very incensed, they remain calm and refuse to deal with the anger that is coming in their direction. What is the result of these orientations? Mountainview Bible Church is not living consistent with its name!

How should Christians respond? First and foremost, Christians need to be familiar with the biblical data on anger. Whether it is God's experience of anger or its presence between individuals, the term "anger" is utilized 390 times in the New International Version of the biblical record. This is filled out even further by terms like "wrath" (197 times), "provoke" (52 times), and "vengeance" (32 times). Immersion in this teaching will prove invaluable for the understanding and managing of one's own anger, as well as the development of appropriate strategies for dealing with others' struggles in this area.

Does God Get Angry?

The phrase that best captures God's anger is "wrath of God." This is not a fashionable teaching in many contemporary churches because it appears, at least to us, to be in marked contrast to God's love. As a result we have a natural propensity to favor the latter and downplay the former. However, these two attributes of God need to be seen in tandem. It is because God loves and cares for us that he reacts with wrath when his people sin against him and break his covenant. In fact, the wilderness experience of the people of Israel reflects this reaction.

Friends or Foes?

> The LORD's anger burned against Israel and he made them wander in the desert forty years, until the whole generation of those who had done evil in his sight was gone. (Num. 32:13)

The prophetic image of the day of the Lord takes the concept of God's wrath even further. It is a warning not just to Israel but to all nations that divine anger will not be spared.

> The great day of the LORD is near—near and coming quickly. Listen! The cry on the day of the LORD will be bitter, the shouting of the warrior there. That day will be a day of wrath. (Zeph. 1:14–15a)

Because of our own experience, we tend to project human qualities onto God and assume that his anger is like our children's temper tantrums in that it is uncontrolled and contains no love or mercy. But God is compassionate and patient. In fact, the Hebrew word for patient literally means "length of wrath." And so these divine attributes blend together.

> The LORD is compassionate and gracious, slow to anger, abounding in love. He will not always accuse, nor will he harbor his anger forever. (Ps. 103:8–9)

This Old Testament theme is picked up in the New Testament when God's anger is placed in contrast to eternal life and the gospel.

> Whoever believes in the Son has eternal life, but whoever rejects the Son will not see life, for God's wrath remains on him. (John 3:36)

> Since we have now been justified by his blood, how much more shall we be saved from God's wrath through him! (Rom. 5:9)

Humanity in its natural state before God is in sin, and because of that God's wrath is the natural consequence. God hates sin and his holiness will not allow it. The only antidote is eternal life found through a relationship with Jesus Christ, the one who experienced God's wrath on the cross. The gospel, then, has the power to overcome sin and to avert the wrath of God. But what of those who are sinning currently? If God is angry with them, why are they not experiencing it? If God's wrath is on them, why is it not obvious? It almost appears that sin has no consequences at present.

> The wrath of God is being revealed from heaven against all the godlessness and wickedness of men who suppress the truth by their wickedness. . . . Therefore God gave them over in the sinful desires of their hearts to sexual impurity. . . . God gave them over to shameful lusts. . . . he gave them over to a depraved mind. . . . (Rom. 1:18, 24, 26, 28)

The teaching of Romans 1 makes it clear that God's wrath is being revealed at the present time. While it is not the full and complete culmination of his anger, it is being expressed. How? By God allowing people to pursue their own course, their own desires, and their own wishes. God's "hands off" approach to sin is his way of expressing anger and wrath. In giving people over to their own sin, God allows them to experience the natural consequences of the sinful life, consequences that are neither honoring to God nor pleasant for humanity. Ironically, his anger in the present is displayed with a type of passivity, a rather marked contrast to what will happen in the future.

> He, too, will drink of the wine of God's fury, which has been poured full strength into the cup of his wrath. He will be tormented with burning sulfur in the presence of the holy angels and of the Lamb. (Rev. 14:10)

Do People Get Angry at God?

The experience of Jonah is an intriguing example of anger at God because the Creator did not do what the created thought he should do! Jonah had avoided going to Nineveh, but eventually, after a slight detour, he preached the message of impending destruction. God, however, "had compassion and did not bring upon them the destruction he had threatened" (Jonah 3:10). Jonah was angry to the point that he asked God to take his life. God's question to him is a penetrating one: "Have you any right to be angry?" (Jonah 4:4) and he follows it up by teaching him the contrast between divine compassion and that experienced by Jonah.

Although the word "anger" is not used, it is clear that Job's communication with God is filled with this kind of feeling. He cannot understand why God is allowing this experience and he expresses himself with poignant feeling.

> I cry out to you, O God, but you do not answer; I stand up, but you merely look at me. You turn on me ruthlessly; with the might of your hand you attack me. (Job 30:20–21)

The psalmist has a similar experience as he struggles with the prosperity of the wicked. The word is not used, but his sentiments seem to reflect an underlying frustration and anger.

> They have no struggles; their bodies are healthy and strong. They are free from the burdens common to man; they are not plagued by human ills. . . . Surely in vain I have kept my heart pure; in vain have I washed my hands in innocence. (Ps. 73:4–5, 13)

A similar sentiment is expressed when David experiences God being distant.

Why, O LORD, do you stand far off? Why do you hide yourself in times of trouble? (Ps. 10:1)

What Does the Old Testament Say about Anger?

There are a number of words for anger, wrath, and fury in the Old Testament. *Anaph* means to snort or blow through the nostrils and is used to describe God's anger. This is the word that the psalmist uses in Psalm 2:12: "Kiss the Son, lest he be angry and you be destroyed in your way." Almost all the uses of this word refer to the nature of God's anger.

Charah and its derivatives communicate a type of anger that is burning, heated, or passionate. Interestingly, this physiologically oriented description of anger is linked with God and humans. It is the word that is used to describe Jonah's anger at God (Jonah 4:1, 4, 9), as well as Nehemiah's anger at the social injustice that God's people were experiencing (Neh. 5:6).

Qatsaph is linked with a sense of wroth or displeasure with others. It is used to describe Moses' anger at Eleazar and Ithamar when they burned the goat in the sin offering (Lev. 10:16).

Provocation and sadness is communicated by the word *kaas*. It is the word used in Proverbs 12:16: "A fool shows his annoyance at once, but a prudent man overlooks an insult."

The Proverbs provide wisdom on the topic of human anger. These verses reflect the dangers that are inherent in poorly managed anger:

> A wise man fears the LORD and shuns evil, but a fool is hot-headed and reckless. (14:16)
>
> A quick-tempered man does foolish things, and a crafty man is hated. (14:17)

A patient man has great understanding, but a quick-tempered man displays folly. (14:29)

A gentle answer turns away wrath, but a harsh word stirs up anger. (15:1)

A hot-tempered man stirs up dissension, but a patient man calms a quarrel. (15:18)

A man of knowledge uses words with restraint, and a man of understanding is even-tempered. (17:27)

A hot-tempered man must pay the penalty; if you rescue him, you will have to do it again. (19:19)

Do not make friends with a hot-tempered man, do not associate with one easily angered, or you may learn his ways and get yourself ensnared. (22:24–25)

A fool gives full vent to his anger, but a wise man keeps himself under control. (29:11)

An angry man stirs up dissension, and a hot-tempered one commits many sins. (29:22)

For as churning the milk produces butter, and as twisting the nose produces blood, so stirring up anger produces strife. (30:33)

What Does the New Testament Say about Anger?

The four main Greek words for anger in the New Testament are *thumos, parorgismos, orge,* and *aganaktesis. Thumos* anger is a turbulent, boiling commotion that can be best illustrated by the lighting of a match. At the point where the match ignites, there is an explosion of the flame. This is *thumos* anger. We experience it as temper or rage. It is referred to in Scripture as "fits of rage" (Gal. 5:20) or "rage" (Eph. 4:31), and is also used to describe God's wrath (Rev. 14:10, 19).[i]

Anger that demonstrates itself in irritation or exasperation is captured in the Greek word *parorgismos*. When Paul is writing to parents in Ephesians he encourages them not to "exasperate your children" (6:4). In other words, do not have a style of discipline that disempowers children and makes them frustrated. To do this is to "embitter" and "discourage" them (Col. 3:21). This is not the boiling, turbulent commotion of *thumos* anger but the internal experience of irritation that occurs in the presence of others' behavior. It was what Paul describes Moses as feeling when he witnessed the idol worship of the people of Israel (Rom. 10:19).[ii]

The third type of anger is of another quality altogether. *Orge* is a settled inner attitude that may, but not necessarily, lead to revenge and personal animosity. This is the most complex of the three words because it can only be understood in its biblical context. For example, when Jesus was going to heal the man with the shriveled hand, the Pharisees were concerned that this was being done on the Sabbath. Jesus "looked around at them in anger [*orge*] and deeply distressed at their stubborn hearts, said to the man, 'Stretch out your hand'" (Mark 3:5). In contrast, Paul admonishes the Ephesian Christians to "get rid of all bitterness, rage [*thumos*] and anger [*orge*], brawling and slander, along with every form of malice" (Eph. 4:31). In the first case, Jesus reacted to religious stubbornness in anger but there was no revenge or personal animosity. In the second case, Paul recognizes that *orge* can move into personal animosity and not reflect a life of righteousness.[iii]

Aganaktesis has the sense of irritation and indignation with a component of grief. When the disciples were not responding well to the children that were being brought to him, Jesus was "indignant" (Mark 10:14). When Paul distinguishes worldly sorrow and godly sorrow in 2 Corinthians 7, he describes the latter as producing "indignation" (v. 11). The emphasis of this word revolves around annoyance at something done by someone else.[iv]

Only used once in the New Testament, *cholao* is connected with the word "gall" in the sense of bitterness of feeling.

Jesus is instructing the Jews and refers to their anger (*cholao*) in healing the man on the Sabbath day (John 7:23).

Is All Anger Sinful?

For many evangelicals there is a fundamental assumption that all anger is wrong and sinful and ought to be purged from our lives. Such a claim may reflect the fact that anger is difficult to manage and control. Also, many people have been on the receiving end of angry outbursts that have left them feeling threatened and intimidated. On the other hand, some of the secular literature on the topic focuses on the validity of human experience, and in the process runs the risk of setting the morality issue aside. For example, in her very helpful book *The Dance of Anger* Harriet Goldhor Lerner says:

> "Is my anger legitimate?" "Do I have a right to be angry?" "What's the use of my getting angry?" "What good will it do?" These questions can be excellent ways of silencing ourselves and shutting off our anger. Let us question these questions. Anger is neither legitimate nor illegitimate, meaningful or pointless. Anger simply is. To ask, "Is my anger legitimate?" is similar to asking, "Do I have a right to be thirsty? After all, I just had a glass of water fifteen minutes ago. Surely my thirst is not legitimate. And besides, what's the point of getting thirsty when I can't get anything to drink now, anyway?" (Lerner, 1985, 3)

In the presence of these two extreme views—one that emphasizes only the sinful component of anger and the other that puts anger into the same moral category as thirst—we need to grapple with the rightness and wrongness of anger.

First, we need to recognize that God experiences anger. It is part of his character. It is one of his attributes. His capacity to react to the sin of others is resident in who he is. Jesus demonstrated that in his pilgrimage on earth. He was not immune from the intense experience of anger, nor was he unwilling to express it. While the term "anger" is not utilized in John 2:12–16, it is clear that when Jesus made a whip out of cords, drove the money changers and their animals out of the temple, and turned their tables upside down, he was experiencing an intense experience of frustration and anger. When you read the words, "Get these out of here! How dare you turn my Father's house into a market!" (John 2:16), you can hear deep passion over a value that has been violated.

Is it possible that our human experience of anger reflects the image of God in us? The fact that we are able to react with passion and candor in the presence of sin and wrongdoing may be traceable to divine qualities. On the other hand, our tendency toward passivity and lack of expression, particularly in the face of others' actions, may reflect our lack of spiritual and psychological sensitivity.

The biblical record does not condemn all anger as sin, nor does it affirm all anger as valid and acceptable. The clearest statement on this issue is found in Ephesians 4:26–27.

> "In your anger do not sin": Do not let the sun go down while you are still angry, and do not give the devil a foothold.

The first phrase communicates a distinction between being angry and sinning. On the one hand, you can be angry, while on the other, you can sin or not sin in that state. The meaning of this becomes much clearer when we understand that Paul uses the word *orge*. In your *orge* anger, an anger that is characterized by a settled inner attitude, do not sin. In other words, this anger, which has the potential for revenge and personal animosity, can turn into sin. It is not the feeling of anger that is the problem here; it is what you do with it. The sin is linked more with personal animosity and vengeance than anger.

Some couples have taken the next phrase and turned it into an injunction to stay up late to resolve their marital squabbles! The argument is simple. The Bible says you should not let the sun go down on your wrath. So we should not go to sleep until we have resolved all of our feelings of anger. Clarifying and moving on from conflict is hard enough, but this so-called biblical injunction adds further pressure. But this is not what Paul is driving at in the passage. We need to recognize that a different word for anger is employed in the second phrase. The anger that is linked with the sun going down is *parorgismos*. It is not that all conflicts need to be resolved before bed, but that the nurturing of *orge* anger may turn it into *parorgismos*. Appropriate anger may turn into sin by the cultivation of the feelings that will precipitate irritation and exasperation and eventually evolve into bitterness.

The final phrase in these two verses—"and do not give the devil a foothold"—can almost seem like an afterthought that is unrelated to what preceded it. However, these three phrases are very much intertwined. If anger moves into sin through a nurturing process that creates irritation and exasperation with resultant bitterness, we are giving the devil an inroad into our lives. In contemporary evangelical thinking, there is a significant amount of discussion about the role of the demonic. In this context, the biblical record links the demonic with how one manages their anger. The word used to describe this process is "foothold."

When we used to play squash, both of us tried to utilize the T-line to our advantage. The T-line is located about three-quarters of the way back in the court. If you stay close to that line, you are able to run to almost any spot on the court without difficulty. On the other hand, if you can get your opponent off the T-line you can drop a shot in the opposite end of the court so he has trouble returning it. Fundamentally, each player needs to be committed to staying close to the T-line. To move away from it is to give your fellow competitor a "foothold." This is precisely what Paul is describing in this passage. If you do not handle anger properly, you are moving away from the T-line and giving the devil an opportunity to make a point.

These two verses provide the touchstone for all the biblical material on anger. To conclude that anger is wrong and sinful is only partially accurate. Depending on the situation that provokes it and the disposition of the person experiencing it, anger may be righteous or it may be sinful.

Where Does Forgiveness Fit In?

The link between forgiveness and anger is an important one, and our understanding of it is rooted in our understanding of God's forgiveness. We have already established that God's wrath abides on those who have not experienced his forgiveness. In contrast, forgiveness leads to a substantially different experience.

> Blessed is he whose transgressions are forgiven, whose sins are covered. Blessed is the man whose sin the LORD does not count against him and in whose spirit is no deceit. (Ps. 32:1–2)

When Nathan confronted David over his sin with Bathsheba and Uriah, the king was seemingly oblivious to all that had happened. But when the truth did sink in and he became aware of the consequences of his behavior, he was able to go through a period of mourning and repentance and then enter into a fresh sense of forgiveness. The forgiveness, as enunciated in Psalm 32, was characterized by four qualities:

1. Forgiveness is a divine response that is resident in God, not in the individual's behavior. Sin demands justice and payment. If God had given David what he deserved, forgiveness would never have been granted.
2. A lack of forgiveness is demonstrated in holding the sin against the other person. They may be reminded of it directly or it may be nurtured in the mind of the offended party. Forgiveness covers the sin so that it is not held against the person. Both literally and metaphorically, it is covered.
3. True forgiveness means that the forensic issues are dealt with. A forgiven person does not have to pay for their sin. Judicially, they stand before God with a sense of being justified, cleared, and as "good as new." They can rest in the assurance that their past sins will not be counted against them.
4. Forgiveness is also motivating and cleansing. When the psalmist describes himself as experiencing an absence of deceit in his spirit, he is capturing the results of being forgiven. There is no longer a need to hide and cover up due to a fear of being caught or punished. Genuine transparency can occur both within and without because the sins of the past have been resolved. This cleansing then becomes a motivator to live with integrity before God.

What does all of this have to do with anger? Let's reflect on the case of Judy. Her eight-year-old daughter was killed in a car accident after they were hit by a drunk driver. These events provoke many emotional reactions, with anger being one of the most dominant. How does Judy deal with her anger? How does it tie to forgiveness? Can she forgive and forget? First, we need to assert that the presence of normal brain functioning makes it impossible to forget. Judy will always remember that fateful day until the day she dies. To ask her not to remember it is to request a physiologically impossible task. As long as we have a memory, most events, particularly the significant ones, will be accessible to us.

Does it make sense that Judy is angry? Her sense of injustice, loss, grief, trauma, and betrayal will be great. We should expect her initial response to be one of anger. She will find it easy to demand justice and payment. Vengeance will be a natural by-product and she will want to hold the drunk driver's sin against him. She will find it natural to make him accountable to her, rather than seeing him as accountable to God, and in the process she will experience an emotional block inside that will defile her spirit. But the question is: Will she be able to get to the place of forgiving the drunk driver?

At times, well-intentioned Christians will advise people like Judy, shortly after an event like this, to write a letter to the drunk driver and tell him she has forgiven him. If she is still numb from the experience, she may find it easy to be compliant and people will be pleased that she has come through such a horrendous time and has forgiven in spite of it. However, until she has experienced the full impact of his sin, she will not be able to grant true forgiveness. The depth of forgiveness is understood best through an appreciation of the depth of sin. Often this can only occur with the mediating role of anger. God's forgiveness of us is the best example of this.

The horrific nature of Calvary is a testament to the horror of sin. Calvary is not a minimization or trivialization of sin. It is not a form of cheap forgiveness. Calvary is not simply a special event that made it possible for us to go to heaven. Rather, it is the full display of God's wrath against our sin. Paul captures this in Galatians when he argues that:

Friends or Foes?

"Cursed is everyone who does not continue to do everything written in the Book of the Law. ". . . Christ redeemed us from the curse of the law by becoming a curse for us, for it is written: "Cursed is everyone who is hung on a tree." (Gal. 3:10,13)

Christ's death and the resultant forgiveness flowed out of God's anger at sin, an anger that was displayed at his Son on the cross. Anger and forgiveness were not separated, but the former was needed in order to get to the latter. God's love and his justice were blended perfectly to accomplish our salvation. Calvary is not just a statement about forgiveness; it is a loud statement on sin.

To accomplish what needs to occur in her healing process, Judy needs to experience the impact of her loss. In that experience, anger will come to the surface. Her natural response will be to want justice and payment and vengeance. She will want to make the driver accountable to her. But in that struggle she will need to come to understand the freeing nature of forgiveness. The wound will not go away, but the poison coming out of it will cease. The accident will always be present, but the emotional trauma that goes with it will subside.

Does this happen all at once? Normally forgiveness has three components. There is the moment of forgiveness that comes after a process of anger and frustration, which has taught us the full impact of the event. Then there is the ongoing work that is required to still live consistent with the forgiveness that has been granted. Forgiveness demands that we respond appropriately to the other party and make a behavioral commitment to demonstrate the love of Christ. Finally, there is the recognition that our existence in the body at present renders all our moral choices to be influenced by sin and frailty. Only in our future heavenly state will we be able to fully, completely, and absolutely give and receive forgiveness. Until then we live between Christ's first and second advent, recognizing that forgiveness is hard work and usually involves an experience of anger.

Christians and Anger—Friends or Foes?

When you think about anger and Mountainview Bible Church, it is probably wise to separate the *way things are* from the *way things should be*. A number of people in the church are "friends" with anger. They carry it, live with it, experience it, and at times express it. Anger is a real part of their lives. And by implication, anger is a real issue in the lives of those who live with them. Many of them have learned to cope with others' anger by tolerating it or denying it. They have allowed the "friendship" to continue.

The biblical record focuses on the *way things should be*. Should Christians be friends with anger or should they see anger as a foe, something to avoid and shun? It depends. The Bible neither presents anger as a righteous response to be pursued, nor as a heinous evil to be removed. Both are options, depending on the person, their attitude, the circumstances, and the ultimate goal. Christians and anger? Maybe friends. Maybe foes.

Personal Reflections

1. Take a closer look at community life in your church. What is the underlying message about anger? Do you have people like William, Sally, Judith, Helmut, Elisabeth, and Tom in the congregation? What impact do these different styles have on other people? How do they affect you? Do you know any of these people well enough to talk with them about their experience of anger?

2. The next time you are angry or upset, think through your experience and expression of anger as you see it by looking at our working definition. Ask yourself some questions:
   a. What emotion is being displayed in the anger?
   b. Can you identify the goal, value, or expectation that has been blocked?
   c. Do you have a sense that your personal worth is being threatened?

   If there is an absence of information in one of these areas, spend more time on it to see if you can understand your anger better. Do not focus on the effect of your anger, only your experience and expression of it.
3. List three things that really upset you at church and another three that upset you in your home environment. Rather than focusing on the trigger that precipitated your anger, zero in on your goals, values, and expectations. What are the goals, values, or expectations that are lurking behind these areas of upset? Go back in your history and see if you can link any of these with early experiences, significant events, particular people, or family themes.
4. Tell someone who knows you well that there are four major ways to express anger—suppression, repression, expression, and confession. Ask him or her which one they see you displaying the most. Talk to someone who knows you less well. Ask him or her the same question. How does this feedback mirror your own self-assessment?
5. As you function in community at your church, which orientation do you tend to fall into most regularly—personality orientation, tolerance orientation, contagious orientation, or denial orientation?
6. Reread the passages in the chapter that talk about the wrath of God. Take a concordance and look up

other references to the same topic. Ask the Lord to give you fresh insight into the relationship between God's wrath and your salvation. Pray that an understanding of the depth of sin will bring a renewed appreciation for the extent of his forgiveness.
7. Jonah, Job, and the psalmist had times in their lives when they were angry with God. Have you ever experienced anger at God? What does that feel like for you? What do you do when you are angry at God?
8. Use a good concordance and/or word study book to trace some of the Old and New Testament words for anger in more depth.
9. Reflect on a recent situation where you were angry. Use the discussion of anger and sin to determine whether your experience and expression of anger were sinful or righteous.
10. Using the definition given in this chapter, think through your current and past relationships and determine if any of them are characterized by a lack of forgiveness. If they are, get the process started so freedom returns to that relationship.

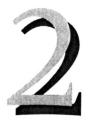

CHARTING A COURSE
EXPLORING YOUR ANGER

> Summary: This chapter begins the adventure of exploring your anger. While there is much to unite us, we are all different in how we respond to situations. Much of that is found in the experience, values, expectations, and goals that we bring to situations. Ultimately, this is traced to our family history as we usually live out many of the historical lessons that we learned. One key aspect of this is the ability to mask our anger both from others and ourselves.

An Adventure in Exploration

Have you ever thought you would like to have been one of the earlier explorers of North America? Can you imagine seeing our eastern coastline for the first time? or cautiously rowing your small craft up some inlet you have never seen? The trees close in on each side. The river current impedes your progress. Uncharted sandbars or contrary current threaten. Perhaps unknown peoples lurk in the shadows of the swamps. You have left the security of your familiar ship anchored in the harbor. Only a few faithful persons accompany you. Supplies are limited. Every shadow ahead, being unfamiliar, stirs twinges of fear or anxiety. It's scary! On the other hand, it is exciting and stimulating; the adrenaline flows. As the oars dip in and out of the water, your heart beats with both fear and excitement, anxiety and anticipation. What lies ahead?

In the first chapter, we met William, Sally, Judith, Helmut, Elisabeth, and Tom from the Mountainview Bible Church. Each experienced anger in the same context of a morning church service. Yet the experience of each was vastly different. "Frustration," "steamed," "irritation," "anger," "exasperation," and "provocation" were words used to describe their personal response to a similar experience, the church service that Sunday morning. We saw that their experience and expression of the emotion of anger varied significantly. If each of these individuals desired to explore the river of anger that surged through their being that Sunday morning, what would be their response to that exploration? Would the experience be the same or different for each of them? Would not their response to the range of emotions experienced be different for each? Would not each of them focus on different aspects of the adventure?

One might focus on the river current. Another might see the new, exciting vegetation and trees. Yet another might be keenly observant of new animals or birds. And others might be watching carefully for persons lurking in the shadows. Some would be very conscious of their comrades in the boat with them and find comfort in that community of support.

Just as your experience and expression of anger are personal and in some dimensions unique, so the adventure

Exploring Your Anger

of exploring your anger will be personal and unique. One of the exciting things about our being human is the apparent unlimited diversity that we represent. We personalize our experience. We personalize our expressions of ourselves. It is said that there are no two fingerprints or DNA patterns alike. God surely must like diversity and, indeed, he appears to celebrate it.

We have a little more difficulty with it. We have a strong tendency to read our experience into that of others. We attribute our thinking, feeling, assessment, perceptions, and the like to others, and wonder or perhaps get angry that they do not see things as we do. That can be very frustrating.

Remember Sally from the Mountainview Bible Church? She was steamed because the woman directly in front of her kept raising her hands in the worship service. Sally's question: "Why would anyone want to bring so much attention to themselves and disrupt everyone around them?" Raising hands in the service was drawing attention to self and disrupting others. She could not see it as worship, which was very likely the woman's perception. Remember Tom? He was provoked as he ticked off the hymns compared to the choruses tally and the ratio didn't fit his personal preference. Would his tally fit your preference?

We certainly do respond personally! Why does my spouse not see how crucially important it is to be on time, or to hang clothes in the closet rather than on every chair, or put ketchup on the table when we have eggs? Why do my children seem oblivious to the things that upset me and go on tirades about silly things?

Wouldn't you think that such awareness would lead us to humility and caution in imposing our perspective on others? It doesn't seem to, does it? No, in fact, we are more likely to be arrogant or prideful about our superior perspective. We get huffed when people don't see things as we do. How can they be so blind, unaware, lacking in insight, or lacking in intelligence? How prone we are to judge, to critique or evaluate others! Our exploration will have to bring us back to that issue.

Yet, there is another consideration. We are different. But we are all the same! There appears to be a finite limit to the variety of human responses. We experience the same emotions. The emotions of fear, love, anger, loss, loneliness, excitement, and one could go on, are the experience of every person. The stimulus may be different, the expression may be different, but there appears to be a finite range of emotional response.

Hebrews 4:15 is an interesting illustration of this point: "For we do not have a high priest who is unable to sympathize with our weaknesses, but we have one who has been tempted in every way just as we are—yet without sin." The King James Version translates "unable to sympathize" as "cannot be touched." The imagery of being "touched" is appealing. When someone is touched with the same feelings you experience, you are aware of sympathy. And does that ever feel good! When someone's emotional response harmonizes with yours, you will feel understood and feel close to that person. It is at the level of our feeling response to life's experiences that we have the potential to enter into each other's lives in helpful ways. Jesus experienced the whole range of human feelings in response to the experiences that are common to the lives of each of us.

Paul phrases it in slightly different language: "No temptation has seized you except what is common to man" (1 Cor. 10:13). There is a commonalty in our experience as humans on this journey of life. That is, we all have the same range of experiences. We have experienced loss, having needs met, being criticized, being praised, and the like.

The difference between us is in the way that we combine experience and emotion. Just as the six friends we met from Mountainview experienced the same church service, they also had a very different experience. Their emotional response, their intellectual content and processing, and their behavioral and verbal expression of themselves were very different.

Person (P) + Experience (E) = Outcome (O)

It gets confusing, right? Let's break it into three pieces. The central part of the equation is the experience we have. Let's call that E. Our six friends experienced a common experience that morning in church, namely, a worship service. We will not detail the constituent parts of E. The outcome (O) for each of them was very different. The O for each of them was different by virtue of different feelings, thoughts, and behavioral expressions in response to E. To understand O for each of them, we would need to explore their feelings, thoughts, physiological response, and behavior. No doubt we would create a very different picture for each of them.

To make sense of why each person has such a different O in response to the same E, we have to look in a different direction. We must ask: What did each of them bring to the encounter with E that morning? They brought their previous experience, personal values, expectations, goals, and their personal identity. One's personal identity is composed of a complex bundle of things, including our sense of worth or significance, our strengths, gifts, abilities, insecurities, our bonding with others, and, generally, how we perceive ourselves. In sum, everyone brought themselves as a person (P).

When we experience E, we are immediately conscious of O and assume O is caused by E. However, the reality is that O may be much more determined by P than by E. In fact, E may only be a trigger to activate O, which will be fueled by P without us or the other person being aware of it.

Joe and Jackie were traveling along the highway discussing the exciting weekend that their young adult group had experienced at a rather exotic campground. The ministry they had experienced had touched each of them rather dramatically. God was real, more real than they had previously experienced. They both caught a fresh vision of the potential for missionary ministry and they were excited about the opportunity to serve God. Suddenly, they became startlingly aware of flashing lights as a police cruiser bore down on them signaling them to stop immediately. Joe, who was driving, jumped on the brakes, his heart pounding, his hands sweating, and beads of perspiration appearing on his forehead as he suddenly realized he was far exceeding the speed limit. He banged the steering wheel with his fist and let out a rather undesirable exclamation. His throat tightened in fear. He saw in his rearview mirror a stern, white officer frowning and then aggressively coming toward the car with his hand close to his gun.

Jackie's response was one of surprise and then fear as she anticipated the police officer coming to their car. Her first thought was that something dreadful had happened at home. Her mother was going into the hospital for some tests the day after they left for the camp. Had something untoward happened? She saw a rather friendly policeman exit his car and approach theirs.

Joe and Jackie had the same experience, but a quite different response. The physiological response of their bodies differed because of their differing perceptions. Their emotional, cognitive, and behavioral responses were quite dramatically different. One significant difference was that one was the driver and the other was not. More important, however, was what they each brought to the situation. Jackie had never been stopped by the police and her perception of a police officer was shaped by a good-natured and jovial uncle who served on the police force in a nearby town. She had lots of contact with the police, all of which was positive.

Joe, on the other hand, saw the police as people to be feared. As a black youth, his culture and his experience told him that the police were often more strict and aggressive with black persons. A ticket would get him in great trouble with his father, who had not been very anxious to loan him the car anyway. How could he be so stupid as to not check his speed? He had always been told that his mind wandered and that he couldn't do two things at once. He was condemned by his mind long before the policeman ever reached the car door.

We understand our experience and expression of anger only as we are prepared to acknowledge our own personal, individualized response in physiology, feeling, thoughts, and behavior, and as we know and accept what we bring to the event as provoking our anger. Another person can only understand our anger if they have the same knowledge. Their knowledge will be based upon our capacity to disclose that information and their ability to receive it. Our knowledge or our ability to disclose may be very deficient. On the other hand, the other person's ability to receive and to comprehend that information may be limited.

Jackie had no awareness of Joe's experience with police officers. He had no knowledge of her background either. She thought his response was irrational and absurd. However, the question is not whether Joe's assessment of himself or the police is based on reality. To him, it is very powerful. Past experience may couple with intuition or imagination to project into a present experience interpretation, attributions, or assessments that are starkly real to the individual, but may make little sense to an observer. Jackie will only understand Joe's reactions to the extent to which she can enter into his experience and to the extent to which he can disclose his experience to her.

Discovery through Exploring Your Anger

Don your pith helmet! We are about to leave the ship, take to the smaller craft, and explore the new continent.

The name of this continent is "Your Anger." It will take courage. There will be dangers. Exploring the unknown is often frightening. We will be armed with the comfort of each other's presence. Let's hold hands. We are committed to seeing this experience through and seeing it through together. We have prayed that the Lord, the great Shepherd, our Guide will lead us and keep us safe.

Have you approached land from a large body of water? The coast seems impenetrable. There seems to be no way in. Sometimes approaching the study of our anger feels like that. Yet as we get closer to the coast, bays, inlets, rivers, and individual trees become distinguishable, and we see the ribbon of water that will take us into the interior. So it is with anger. Anger wears many disguises, masks that hide what is behind it. Often those masks are characterizations—frightening, hideous, or joyful, funny or serious and stern. But usually the anger is rooted in our history and will display itself in either implosive or explosive ways.

Anger: The Fruit from a Family Tree

Do you remember the story of Jacob and his family in the Bible? You may wish to refresh your memory by reading chapters 24 through 50 of the Book of Genesis. Jacob was the son of Isaac and Rebekah, the grandson of Abraham, the man of faith. You can trace the experience and expression of anger in that family tree. Beginning with the hatred between Esau and Jacob, we have the story of a truly dysfunctional family, ending with the death of Joseph. Jacob expressed his anger toward Esau, and later in his relationship with his father-in-law Laban. Do you suppose there was a relationship between the anger of Jacob and that of his sons toward Joseph, which led to his being sold into slavery in Egypt? Undoubtedly!

Anger is one of the fruits that grows in family trees. You have heard the phrase "Like father, like son." Unfortunately, anger is learned in families. Sometimes children learn to get their way through anger expression. The selectivity that occurs in the expression of anger is learned. Have you ever thought about how much control we exercise in expressing our anger? We select our means and ways, and we select the objects of our anger, often with great consistency.

Tom and Elizabeth came for counseling, both concerned about Tom's anger. Elizabeth said her main complaint was Tom's "wood swearing" at every provocation. What is wood swearing? Tom looked at the floor sheepishly as Elizabeth explained. Apparently, when angry Tom would not raise his voice at her or the children, nor did he ever hit anyone. However, he went throughout the house slamming door after door with great gusto! That, Elizabeth said, was wood swearing. Tom was very selective, very controlled. The variety of ways to express anger must be nearly infinite, but we are selective and we do exercise control in that selection.

Both of us have worked with delinquent youth. They, too, were selective. Some always focused their anger toward the destruction of property. Others would attack individuals. Some were only verbal and could excel in that department. Selection and control. How do you exercise control? You may feel out of control, but very likely you are controlled. In your analysis of your anger, look for the consistency of expression that indicates control.

Anger: Implosion or Explosion

Anger may be expressed in two directions: inward or outward. We call anger expressed inward, toward the self, *imploding anger.* This bursting of anger inward, toward the self, may involve what is usually referred to as repression or suppression, as discussed in chapter 1. The physiological aspects of anger will be evident in the body, and the anger will express itself in feelings, thoughts, and behavior.

Otherwise, we may experience *exploding anger,* which is the bursting of anger outward, being directed toward others, God, or things. This is often referred to as expression, letting it out or venting the emotions. It will often be seen as temper or aggression.

Understanding the Masks of Anger

Masks serve a purpose. Have you seen a Shakespearean play or another play that employed masks? Masks cover. Masks may exaggerate. Masks may deceive. Masks may protect. Masks may frighten or entice. Perhaps there is an element of the dramatic in each of us because we all have a tendency to use masks. Children are less likely to use masks. As we grow older, we seem to develop masking as a way of relating to the world and others.

Masks are used with intentionality. The many masks we use in our expression of anger are instrumental. That is, they accomplish a purpose. The mask is intended to accomplish the intention of the anger that it is hiding. Before we look at the masks we use to cover anger, we need to acknowledge that anger itself may be a mask. Also, we need to explore briefly a framework for looking at anger and explore our family's expression of anger.

George could get angry very quickly. He was a large man, but did not feel he had good verbal skills. He loved his daughter and two grandchildren who had been abandoned by a husband who just disappeared. He was getting up in years, but in his opinion he now had to support his daughter, although advice was about all he had to offer. Susan was tiny like her mother, just a hair over five feet tall. She had a good job and was supporting herself and her children quite well. She did feel lonely and inadequate in making many decisions. When she asked her dad for advice, he was free to give it and she appreciated that. However, if she had a different idea he would fly into a rage. It was an awful and a frightening sight. He walked about in his anger. He blustered and would go red in the face. He would peer over his glasses and hover over her as he gestured in frustration. He shouted to make his point. Susan felt intimidated, small, in fact, like a little child being reprimanded. She would cower into the chesterfield chair and wait for things to abate.

George's anger was a mask. His heart was breaking for his daughter. His compassion for his grandchildren was great. His desire for vengeance against his son-in-law was a powerful force. His sense of inadequacy was deep. Verbiage with which to articulate his thoughts was absent. His values of loyalty, commitment, honesty, and integrity were breached by his son-in-law, but he was unaware of this source of his anger. His expectations that men should care for their children were breached. All of these things were masked by anger.

Anger may be masked by imploding upon one's self. When anger bursts inward it may be expressed as malice toward self, or expressions of unworthiness, shame, guilt, or any form of putting one's self down. Sometimes it is safer to cover one's anger toward others by berating or beating one's self. In fact, sometimes when I humiliate myself, I gain sympathy, consolation, or a change of behavior on the part of the person I am angry toward. I may do this by isolating myself from others, by overbonding with others, by becoming a doormat, by sabotaging relationships, by rebellion, by immoral behavior that is self-destructing, and so on. We are quite ingenious in covering our anger toward others by self-negation. Sometimes Christian people will use a form of spiritual self-abuse by declaring sinfulness, unworthiness, or abject humility as a means of covering anger, which they do not have freedom to express. It takes a great deal of courage to take an inventory on how we mask anger by this process of imploding upon the self. This may be very destructive, for when we become our own enemy it is difficult to win. The war against one's self is the war that can only be won by losing. One might think of this form of masking anger as emotional blackmail against one's self. It will often manifest itself in depression. Do you have the courage to explore the possibility that you use this mask? Often the person using such a mask needs help to reverse the process because self-abuse is a most devastating form of abuse.

Anger may be masked by a great variety of physiological responses. The physical responses and expression of anger are a function of the autonomic nervous system in its interaction with our glandular system and brain chemistry. Essentially, anger is a state of physiological arousal. This physiological preparedness involves body chemistry, which activates many functions such as heart rate and blood pressure, and involves other bodily changes such as redistribution of the blood supply to muscle systems and vascular changes, which prepare the body for action. When one continues in this state of arousal for lengthy periods, stress is placed upon the body and damage can occur, which may lead to physical pathology and the onset of psychosomatic symptoms. These vary from person to person depending on our physical condition and a variety of genetic factors. Anger is sometimes masked by physiological outcomes such as gastrointestinal complaints, including stomach sensitivity, ulcers, colitis, or similar problems. It is common for people who mask anger to experience a variety of headaches, deficiency in immune system functioning, hypertension, chronic exhaustion or emotional reactions such as depression. One needs to explore the presence of such symptoms to determine if they are masking anger.

Anger may be masked by verbal behavior. Verbal behavior may implode upon one's self and may be expressed in self-negation. Verbal behavior may explode and express itself in bullying verbal behavior, sarcasm (see Job 5:21; 19:2; Pss. 57:4; 64:3; Prov. 12:18, 21), compulsive talk, loud language, or avoidance of meaningful communication. Sometimes people will be quite subtle such as the "I like you but . . ." style, which may give the appearance of niceness followed by the twist of the knife. Again, some cover anger by what they would describe as truth telling, which frequently expresses itself in rigidity, legalism, or exaggeration where anger is covered with a mask of pretended love and concern.

Finally, anger may be masked by various behaviors. These may include habitual lateness, selective inattention, physical posturing, gestures of control or threat, aggressive behaviors, physical withdrawal, or intimidation.

One must be careful in achieving an understanding of one's masks. Be gentle. Be tentative. Walk around the issue and do not rush to conclusions. In counseling you will be assisted in this exploration. Remember that masks are usually protective in nature and one must be cautious and considerate. We often are only free to remove a mask if we feel safe. This often means learning an alternative way to express one's self with more effectiveness.

The Anger Equation

When we experience anger it is often the expression of anger that we focus on, the behavior we have learned to employ in expressing anger. What we would like to do is to explore the experience of anger in terms of the emotions, thoughts, and physiology of anger. Next, we would like to suggest exploring the personal factors that initiate our experience of anger. One could represent this in a diagram such as the one below.

THE ANGER EQUATION

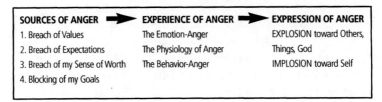

We have suggested the expression of anger is in imploding or exploding behavior, which we fear because it often leads to harm or hurt to self or others. When we fear these expressions, we will often mask the expression in some way to protect ourselves or others from the anger. It is helpful to look at different and more effective ways to express our anger. However, we should first understand the experience of anger and the initiating personal factors that lead to the expression and may inform the expression.

For now, let's acknowledge that anger is an experience of emotions and thoughts and that it is accompanied by physiological responses which we have briefly discussed. We will come back, in later chapters, to discuss the emotions, thoughts, and behaviors in more detail.

Let's look at the personal factors that initiate our experience of anger. Anger occurs when my goals are blocked. I want the traffic to be clear when I go to work. When I get caught in the traffic, I become angry. Anger is often a response to a breach of values. When my sense of justice has been breached, I become angry. When my sense of fairness, honesty, and the like are breached, I become angry. It is interesting to notice in the biblical material covered in the first chapter that God becomes angry when his values are breached. Third, when my expectations are breached I become angry. It may be possible for me to assess my values in the light of God's values. God becomes angry when his expectations are breached, as illustrated in the biblical material. It is more difficult to be clear that my expectations are appropriate and valid. Fourth, when my sense of worth is breached I become angry. If I feel put down, devalued, depreciated, or invalidated in some way, I become angry. God also responds with anger when he is devalued or depreciated by humanity, representing him in idolatry through the worship of created things rather than the Creator.

Often that which activates our anger may be understood as a breach of goals, values, expectations, or our sense of worth. Recognizing that means we can assess the experience of anger and determine whether it is an appropriate response. Then we can ask whether there are more effective ways to express those values than in the behavior by

An Illustration of Nonproductive and Productive Cycles of Anger

A Nonproductive Anger Cycle

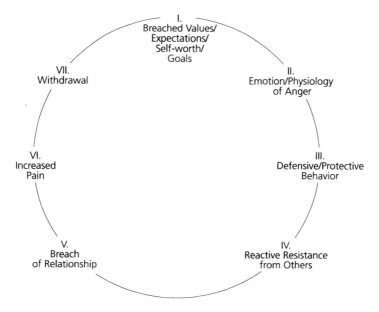

Charting a Course

A Productive Anger Cycle

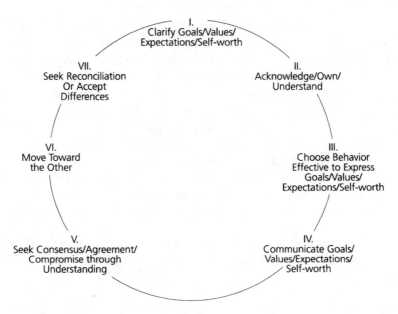

which we have learned to express our anger. We then modify our behavior accordingly.

Mapping the Adventure of Exploration through Pastoral Counseling

Some of us find it helpful to explore troubling emotions like anger with a co-pilgrim—someone who understands the journey, has an appreciation for its complexity, and is willing to walk with us. For those of you who may decide to pursue this kind of help, we would like to introduce some key assumptions of Strategic Pastoral Counseling that will aid your understanding of the process.

We believe that people grow and mature as they move from dependency to increasing self-directedness. This is not a statement about your relationship with the Lord as much as a description of the relationship between a pastor and a parishioner. This means that you are expected to assume considerable responsibility for the process and outcome of the counseling in which you are engaged. People enter into new learning as they are encouraged to identify resources within themselves to see past experiences as a reservoir for learning through experimentation. In counseling, you will be encouraged to find resources within yourself and, if you are married, resources in your spousal relationship. You will also be encouraged to explore past experiences to find patterns of emotional response, thought, and behavior that you may wish to change to more effective ways of responding to your current experience.

Readiness to learn is influenced by embedding learning in the desire for change in social roles. New knowledge does not necessarily lead to new behavior. New understandings must be creatively expressed in behavioral changes that create new patterns of response and expression. Learning will be entered into more readily if learning is associated with problem solving in response to a sense of inadequacy in specific situations. Thus you will be asked to identify areas of difficulty in relationships. The humility to do this is not always easy to come by. The counseling process will bring into focus specific behavior that you desire to change. Understanding the roots of that behavior often enables one to creatively plan change.

One of the ways this specificity and personal responsibility for change will be kept in the forefront will be through the use of homework. Unlike your school experience, you set the curriculum and your life is the textbook. As you look at the textbook of your life, you may come to different and more helpful ways of interpreting the experiences that have shaped you in your development. To continue the image, you will be encouraged to write the next volume of your life with different patterns of behavior, thought, and emotions that you choose to incorporate. Your pastoral counselor will request your engagement in homework that will help to identify and clarify issues and new behaviors.

As you read the following chapters, you will acquire an increasing number of tools with which to work with your anger. The more raw material (your episodes of anger) you have to deal with, the more you will see the value of all the tools and the more skilled you will become in using the tools to better understand. You will learn new ways to express yourself that will be more effective and more honest. You will be able to take the biblical material you discovered in chapter 1 and see how it corresponds to and informs your anger. As you work, pray for the enlightening ministry of the Spirit of God to lead you into the truth that will free you from the negative outcomes you have been experiencing as a result of anger inappropriately understood and expressed.

We hope this will be a real adventure of partnership, where you and your counselor will experience the dynamic work of the Holy Spirit in the healing process.

Personal Reflections

1. Our image for exploring anger has been the early pilgrims arriving on the east coast of North America. Seriously examining the interior of our lives is not an easy task. Tune in to your own experience of exploring anger. What images come to mind? What feelings are you experiencing as you embark on this adventure? What are your fears and anxieties?
2. Sometimes we find out about ourselves by observing others. As you read about the various people at

Mountainview Bible Church, who do you identify with the most? In what ways are your experiences and expression of anger the same? In what ways are they different?
3. Go back to those people again and make some assumptions. What kinds of experiences do you think existed in their respective histories? Did they externalize or internalize their anger? Did their strategy work for them? The goal here is to get in touch with the rich variety we experience as we explore our anger and that of others.
4. We have suggested that pride and humility play a major role in how we deal with our own histories and preferences. It is natural for us to adopt the moral high ground on our own viewpoints and assume everything and everyone else is deficient. Can you think of an area in your life where this perspective on pride and humility makes sense?
5. Think of an illustration of anger in the Bible. Take our "Person (P) + Experience (E) = Outcome (O)" equation and analyze the biblical story through this grid. Seek as much detail and specificity as possible.
6. Jackie thought that Joe's experience of anger was irrational and absurd. Think of a recent situation where you had that reaction to someone else's anger. If you know them well, have a conversation that will help you understand the experiences and expectations that precipitated their response.
7. We would suggest that you explore the fruit on your family tree, especially with respect to anger expression. It takes courage. Be sure to clarify in your mind that in exploring one's family of origin the purpose is not to attribute intention or to assign guilt to any family member. To do either of those things engenders a sense of disloyalty and guilt, which destroys the freedom we need to explore the behavior pat-

terns. Work hard to focus on the behavior manifested and your response to it, not the intention of the other persons. In fact, it is helpful to intentionally attribute acceptable intention or motivation to others while focusing on the behavior and our response to it.

Here is the plan. Look at each family member—father, mother, siblings, and self. How was anger expressed by each? Write it down, making brief notes. When you have completed that task, move to the question of how each responded when anger was expressed by other family members. You have noted the differences in expression; now focus on the differences in response to anger expressed by others. You could be creative and set this up in a chart form. Get as clear a picture as you can. Feel free to consult carefully with others in your family or others who have had opportunity to observe your family. You are doing a nonjudgmental analysis of anger experience and expression in your family of origin. Don't get too serious; we are exploring with tentativeness, not judgment. When we discover something that facilitates our learning, we will know it. We are opening ourselves to explore, with appropriate caution, territory we may not have entered before so let's not jump too quickly to premature conclusions about what we see. Sharing these explorations with your pastoral counselor will help as we seek learning that will facilitate our growth.

8. Is your expression of anger more frequently imploding or exploding? Are you aware of feelings, thoughts, or actions that are directed toward yourself? Or, are you more aware of anger exploding outward toward others, God, or things? Keep a diary of your anger for a few weeks. Simply acknowledge, accept, and catalogue your experiences. In writing the diary your purpose is not to analyze each entry, but to accumu-

late a sufficient number of entries. When you have ten or twelve accounts, then you may reflect on them. Study to see if imploding or exploding was more common. Do you see any patterns?

9. Masks do not just hide us from others, but also keep us out of touch with ourselves. We have talked about masks of implosion, physiology, verbal behavior, and other behaviors. Can you identify your major masks? Are there some you would like to gently remove? Are there some that others might help you identify more carefully?

10. At the end of this chapter we have provided an illustration of nonproductive and productive anger cycles. Pull out a few of your recent anger episodes and try and work them through the cycle, seeking to determine whether they were productive or nonproductive and why.

3

THE POWER OF FEELINGS
SIN OR RIGHTEOUSNESS?

> Summary: The deacons of Mountainview Bible Church have some conflict in their meeting. The chairman lets fly at the group, but eventually things calm down, order is restored, and the meeting is closed in prayer. The anger issues are unresolved until two of the members admit to their feelings, seek to understand them, and work at resolving the broken relationship. The process of acknowledging and accepting our feelings is a prerequisite to determining whether or not they are in harmony with God's will.

A Messy Deacons Meeting

It is 10:26 P.M. on Monday night. Around the boardroom of Mountainview Bible Church sit seven deacons. Garth, the chair, has been at the church the longest. Doreen is the newest deacon, having just come on six months ago. Alex, Mildred, Michael, Alice, and Barry are observing at this point as Garth and Doreen have a rather heated exchange on whether to involve the congregation in decision making about the parking lot expansion. Garth thinks the decision is clear-cut and does not require any more discussion tonight, much less congregational affirmation. Doreen is trying to impress on him the importance of the church owning the project and the fact that the deacons do not have all the understanding. At that point Garth erupts.

"What do you mean, we don't have all the understanding? I have been at this church for thirty-five years and have chaired this group for ten of the last twelve years. Don't tell me that I do not know what I am talking about."

"Garth, I'm not talking about you. I'm talking about church ownership and the importance of the whole body being involved in decision making."

"That's the problem with the younger generation. You get a bunch of liberals in here and they want everything to go to a vote. Whatever happened to old-fashioned leadership?"

"Garth, I wish you would not get so angry about this and we could talk about it calmly. I simply want—"

"Don't instruct me on being calm. As the chair of the deacons I have every right to express my opinion and let the group know what I think."

At this point Alex and Mildred are getting quite uncomfortable. Alex and Garth are friends and he is aware of his tendency to "lose it" in meetings. He is nervous about what might happen next. Mildred hates conflict so she is really struggling to know what to do. She just wishes it would all stop. Alice and Barry had long days at work and both of them begin to look at the clock, wondering if the meeting will ever end. Michael is a peacemaker and decides that he will jump in to resolve the problem, at least as he sees it.

"I think it would be helpful if we could keep feelings out of this and get back to the issues at hand."

Sin or Righteousness?

At this point Garth stands up and bangs his hand on the table.

"I am really tired of all of you not supporting me in my role as chair. Sometimes I feel like longevity in this church is a hazard, not a strength. Those of you who are younger do not seem interested in listening to those who are older."

At that point he turns to walk out of the room and Doreen jumps in.

"Let's just leave it, Garth. I am sorry that I upset you and that you felt undermined. If you think we should make the parking lot decision ourselves, I will be happy to make that motion."

Visibly relieved, Garth sits down, Doreen makes the motion, Michael seconds it, and Garth closes in prayer. In his prayer he thanks God that the group was able to resolve their conflict and that harmony and unity were restored. He thanks God for making this possible. At the end there is a resounding "Amen" from around the table and everyone makes their way to the parking lot.

It is now 12:57 A.M. on Tuesday morning. Garth is lying in bed, awake, beside his wife Dorothy, who was asleep when he got home from the meeting. He is tossing and turning and replaying the last part of the deacons meeting in his mind. He is angry at Doreen and wonders why she was put on the deacons board to begin with. He was never comfortable with her, and he has often wondered if she was out to get him. He has heard rumors that some of her theology is not very evangelical, and he questions if that is what is coming out in the meetings. Apparently a number of people in the church find her pushy.

Doreen is sitting in her condominium living room overlooking the city. She is in her housecoat and is sipping herbal tea. She is in turmoil. She has the heart of the church in mind and desperately wants to serve with this commitment. Tonight she felt bulldozed and she recognizes that this is the same problem that happens at work when someone gets angry at her. It is like her relationship with her father all over again. She expresses her point of view, a strong man uses anger to undercut it, and she sweetly goes along with him. As she thinks, she cries quietly with a sense of sadness and frustration that she cannot express what she is feeling in clearer terms. She wishes that she would not let herself get walked over when she believes she is right. In a way she is angry at herself.

Michael is sound asleep. He came home from the meeting quite happy with the way it had gone. He believes his spiritual gift is giving mercy, so he was pleased that he had another opportunity to bring peace to a conflictual situation. The experience fortified him and gave him a sense of personal well-being. Secretly he is glad that God has placed him on the deacons board because it gives him frequent opportunities to inject harmony into conflict.

Let's revisit our equation: Person (P) + Experience (E) = Outcome (O). Person represents previous experience, personal values, expectations, goals, and personal identity. It is what each individual brings to conflictual situations. Experience represents our response (emotion, thoughts, physiology) to the events under consideration, while outcome is the expression each person manifested in behavior, whether in words or actions.

Garth, Doreen, and Michael experienced the same event (E), a deacons meeting. However, in the meeting and in the wee hours of the next morning there was great diversity in the outcome of that experience. Garth went from the expression of extreme anger in the meeting to a quiet thankful prayer to a disruptive sleep that is focused on Doreen's problems. What did Garth bring to the event that led to that range of emotional responses?

Doreen went from being expressive and assertive to compliant in the meeting, but went home and felt great turmoil. Her focus is on her relationship with her father and the themes that relationship seem to generate. In some ways she is more angry with herself than with Garth. What did Doreen bring to the event that produced those outcomes?

Then there is Michael. When the feelings came to the surface in the meeting, he was very uncomfortable and decided that this problem should be addressed. He is pleased that his statement "Feelings should be kept out of this" led to resolution and a sense of unity. He did not reflect very deeply on all of this, but experienced inner peace that he was able to make a contribution. What did Michael bring to the event that produced these outcomes?

Feelings, Blaming, and Masks

In previous chapters, we have looked at the many aspects of anger. It involves feelings, anger, and will. It has physiological components to it and it can be imploded or exploded. Experientially, however, most of us are aware of the physiological and emotive sides of anger. When Doreen tells Garth to be calm he really loses it, partially because he was so absorbed by the feelings that a decision to "cool it" seems impossible. Imagine trying to speak reason to Garth when he is standing at the edge of the table, banging his hand. If anyone had tried that intervention, the table might have been banged much louder.

The truth is, most of us lead with our feelings when it comes to anger. We are not aware of goals, values, expectations, or self-worth. We are not thinking that one of them has been blocked. We are just aware that we are mad! But we do need to take this a step further if we are going to understand and resolve the problem of anger. Let's do that by asking this question: Who is furthest ahead in understanding the reality of what happened?

Before we answer that question, look at Garth. He is lying in bed blaming Doreen for what happened. He had done the same thing in the meeting. She was:

telling him he did not know what he was talking about.

part of the younger generation that was a bunch of liberals.

like the others, not supporting him in his role as chair.

part of a younger group that did not listen to the older people.

That is very typical when we are angry. Listen to some of the phrases that we use when we are angry:

"She makes my blood boil!"
"He gets under my skin!"
"Every time I see him I get furious!"
"I find my dad infuriating!"

All of these phrases allocate blame and fault elsewhere. Someone else has created/caused/facilitated my anger, and I am not responsible. All of these phrases express deep feeling, but there is no personal accountability for those feelings. That is Garth's state, and it is unlikely that he will move beyond it if he maintains his "Doreen is to blame" game.

The corollary to the "blame game" approach in anger is to ignore any of the stimuli that may have precipitated it and to communicate that others do not have a right to be angry and should stop feeling it. In a sense that was Michael's position. He intervened when the feelings got intense and invited both participants to shut their feelings down. For him the expression of anger was not appropriate, and peace was defined as the complete absence of anger. Although he does not realize it, his "ministry" in the meeting managed to turn off the tap, but it did not turn off the main valve. As soon as Garth and Doreen got home the tap got turned on again.

It is important to note that both approaches ignore the personal feeling. In the first case, Garth is not focused on

Sin or Righteousness?

what he is experiencing. He is going through mental gymnastics to paint Doreen into a corner that she will never get out of. As long as he dwells on what she is like, he will be oblivious to what he is experiencing. In the second scenario, the feelings have been wiped out completely and there is a niceness in the air. Everyone seems to be happy, the prayers are sweet, but the emotions still linger.

It would appear that Doreen is dealing with reality. She is focusing on her own feelings and history and a recurrent theme that rears its head in other contexts. She has not adopted Garth's blaming style, nor is she into the denial of Michael. In a sense, she is the healthiest because her commitment to understand the way things are is the greatest.

Two key questions need to be asked. What is Garth feeling? and why is he angry? Can Garth and Doreen talk about their experience at the meeting without holding each other responsible?

The next morning Garth wakes up and his wife Dorothy asks him how the meeting went. Initially he starts to lash into Doreen and what she is like, but Dorothy interrupts him.

"You sound really angry. Were you like that in the meeting?"

"I guess I was. Do I sound that bad?"

"Yes, this sounds like the night they voted you off that committee at the club. Do you remember that?"

"I remember being royally ticked, but I guess this one seemed different, at least last night."

"Are you back into the 'no one wants me, I'm not good for anything' space?"

(Quietly) "Yeah."

In a very short time Garth has become aware not only of the depth of feeling, but also some of the thoughts lurking behind those feelings. After his company downsized and he was released, he went through a painful stage of insecurity, feeling that his age was a real hazard. He was replaced by a much younger woman who had significantly more education, but less experience. His sense of personal identity, which up until that point had been wrapped up in his work, took a real beating. Since that time he has been hypersensitive to "being included" and "belonging," particularly from younger females. Any time he was confronted or even questioned, his back went up and he experienced anger. In many ways that was what he went through last night. His personal worth was threatened and he went on the attack. Unfortunately, Doreen bore the brunt of it. The next step was clear.

"Doreen? It's Garth. I was hoping I would get you before you went to work. Is this a good time to talk?"

"Yes, it's fine."

"First of all I want to apologize for last night. It may sound strange to you, but I was not aware of how angry I was until this morning. I realize that there are a lot of other things going on for me and you ended up taking the brunt of my anger. The truth is, I'm not even sure my anger was about the parking lot. It was more about my own sense of security and well-being. It's the retirement thing rearing its ugly head again."

"Garth, I really appreciate your apology. I remember you talking about your pain over retirement a few meetings back and I know it has been a tough struggle for you. I accept your apology and really value what you just said. I did a lot of thinking about last night too, and I realize that I have some personal issues to deal with as well. I think the incident brought some historical themes to the surface for me. In fact, it left me feeling more angry with myself than at you!"

(With a laugh) "Wow, both me and you angry at you. That's a lot!"

Do you notice the difference between the next morning and the night before? The feelings of anger have not been denied or explained away. Garth did not say, "Doreen, I was having a bad day yesterday and did not come across very well at the meeting." Doreen did not say, "No problem, Garth, forgiven and forgotten." Both of them acknowledged the feeling of anger. But, most importantly, they took full responsibility for that anger and did not blame the other person. Garth did not go into all the details, but was willing to share that there were "a lot of other things going on" for him and that this contributed to the anger he was experiencing. Similarly, Doreen admitted that "some historical themes" came to the surface for her. Both of them went away from the telephone conversation with greater understanding of themselves and each other, rather than with a catalogue of negative qualities in the other person that caused their anger. They were only able to do this because they could admit to the feelings of anger.

Unfortunately, there are a lot of confusing messages about feelings in Christian circles, which have created difficulty for many people. In fact, many Christians are told that they are not supposed to go with their feelings. Feelings cannot be trusted. In some quarters this has almost become a theological reality: we should start with faith, then move to facts, and let the feelings follow after. That seems to make feelings unimportant, almost insignificant. In the current situation, an awareness of feelings brought Garth closer to confronting the truth of what was going on. When he was out of touch with his feelings, his rage against Doreen persisted.

We like to use three terms to help people understand this area: acknowledge, accept, and approve. First, it is very important to acknowledge that we have feelings. If we are not honest with ourselves before God, we are missing what is actually happening. To acknowledge feelings is really to describe reality: This is the way things are right now. The next step is to accept what we are feeling. Often people will acknowledge in a grudging way that they are experiencing emotion, but will have trouble accepting particular feelings. This is particularly true with anger. Some people can acknowledge that they are having feelings, but do not accept the fact that they are angry. Somehow anger is not right. It is sinful and unacceptable.

Accepting that you are angry is not a statement about whether or not you approve of your anger. For example, to accept the fact that you sin does not mean you approve of it. Before we came to faith in Christ, we had to accept the fact that we were enemies of God. That was a necessary first step before we could repent of our sin and come to Christ. To accept that you are angry is only to say: This is the way things are right now. This kind of acceptance requires an integrity and an authenticity that describes reality for what it is. Having done that, you are ready to reflect on the area of sin and righteousness, or in the language that we have been using, you are ready to decide if you approve or disapprove of the way things are. In essence, this describes what happened to Garth. In acknowledging and accepting his angry feelings, he was able to move quickly to the place where he realized they were inappropriate and to request forgiveness. In many, maybe most, situations it is not that easy, but the principle is an important one.

In contrast, Michael has trouble acknowledging that he has feelings and would prefer that others not express their emotions either. When anger does come, he tries to downplay it and deny it. He can put on a happy face and grin and bear it. In a sense, he does not allow himself to experience anger because he does not want to feel. Careful reflection on his history and family dynamics reveals a strong threefold rule: don't feel; avoid conflict; keep things happy. Ironically, the absence of acknowledgment and acceptance makes it very difficult for him to deal with the approval question. He does not have to wrestle with the moral questions around anger because anger is not allowed in his world. It is significant that his family background gets in the way of his ability to confront biblical realities.

Sin or Righteousness?

You can imagine Michael's surprise at the next deacons meeting when Garth describes his own experience after the meeting, and both he and Doreen share what happened in their phone conversation.

"But I thought everything was resolved in the meeting. You closed with a very moving prayer about unity and peace and the fact that God had worked his purposes through the conflict."

"Michael, I did not do that insincerely, but I realized later on that night that my feelings of anger and frustration did not disappear with the prayer. In an odd sense, the prayer helped to keep them underground."

Garth illustrates the power of the masks that we discussed in the previous chapter. Remember that masks can cover, exaggerate, deceive, and accomplish a purpose. In this case, the pious prayer at the end of the meeting facilitated Garth's unconscious desire to cover his inner issues on anger. It also exaggerated a spiritual veneer that on the surface appeared to have depth and conviction. But in the process it was deceptive because it masked the truth. Reality took second place to appearance, with the intended purpose of smoothing the waters and not having to deal with conflict. Paradoxically, Garth's mask was a perfect fit with Michael's family rules.

For Christians there are usually two types of spiritual masks. The first one that Garth illustrates is the "denial of anger" mask. In this case the mask keeps up the good front. The person is congenial, speaking with warm Christian words, but underneath there is a minor volcano that is desperately trying to erupt. It is this process that keeps many people sleepless after meetings at the church. During the meeting they put on the serene "I'm not angry" mask, but the mask falls off when they hit the parking lot and they are forced to confront the feeling. Keep in mind that this process is often, although not always, outside of conscious awareness.

The other spiritual mask does not hide anger, but expresses it with great passion. Do you remember Tom at Mountainview Bible Church? His Sunday morning responsibility was determining the ratio of choruses to hymns. When he interacts with William after the service, he is talking about worship, a topic that ties to Scripture and the core of our spirituality. His communication is angry and intense and he appears to have a lot of passion about worship. At one level you could say that Tom is being biblical because he is talking about a biblical theme. But his behavior in the church is hardly reflective of a godly man who is seeking to do what is right. He is harboring bitter attitudes towards those at the front, and much of it relates to his own preferences which he has absolutized. Fundamentally, there is a lot of pride at the core, combined with legalism, hostility, rigidity, criticism, and aggression. However, his mask of "I'm interested in the Bible and the priority of worship" hides that core, both to him and to many people he talks to.

We talked earlier about the importance of being cautious and considerate with masks. People will only remove their masks if they feel safe and if they have learned an alternative way to express themselves. Notice, Garth was able to drop his mask the next morning when he was able to receive his wife's gentle prodding. If someone had confronted him in the meeting, he probably would have become more entrenched in his anger.

The "Toms" of the evangelical world are more difficult to deal with. One of the major problems with self-righteousness is its inherent deception. Self-righteous people do not explicitly say, "I'm better than everyone else and my preferences and experience must be followed by all who are in my church." To say that would be to admit arrogance, a statement most would avoid. What self-righteous people will do very often is put on the "I'm very concerned; I'm very upset" mask, throw in a great array of Bible verses, and communicate with biblical jargon.

It is mandatory that you have a relationship with the "Toms" before the mask will come down. It is also important that your own feelings are kept in check as you interact. "Toms" can be extremely irritating in their picky obsessiveness. They often have a verse for everything or some kind of spiritual platitude. An awareness of the tenor and thrust of Scripture is extremely valuable in these situations so the "proof-texting" style submits to the bigger picture. Finally, genuine care and compassion is mandatory. No one is going to drop the spiritual veneer mask and expose their arrogance unless they feel safe, valued, and have a sense that there is a healthy alternative.

Grappling with Scripture

When we get into the realm of approval, we are really asking two questions. Does God approve of the anger? Do I approve of the anger? Part of our struggle as Christians is to achieve harmony between the answers to these two questions. If God sees our anger as sinful, then we need to repent of it and strive against it. On the other hand, if God does not disapprove of our anger, then we should not beat ourselves up over it. Those who have trouble acknowledging feelings do not even think about the sin and righteousness question. They are so concerned to deny what they are feeling that the morality side of it is relatively unimportant. The thoughtful Christian acknowledges and seeks to understand the feelings that are being expressed, but the emotional side does not become the moral touchstone. Rather, morality needs to be understood with reference to biblical data.

First, it is important to realize that the Bible does not say that all anger is right or wrong. It really depends on the passage that we are looking at and the situation that is under consideration. It is interesting that God asked Jonah if he had any right to be angry. In that situation it appears that God was unhappy with Jonah's emotional expression. Jonah was frustrated because God had been compassionate and had not brought the destruction on Nineveh that he had promised. In contrast, you have Paul's words in 2 Corinthians 7. He is encouraging the Corinthians to engage in godly sorrow, a quality that is characterized by indignation, alarm, concern, and a readiness to see justice done. Interestingly, the word he uses for indignation is a word that is in the "angry" family and means irritation. Here Paul is praising this kind of emotive response. In Ephesians 6, Paul, in talking about parental responsibilities toward children, warns that parents should not exasperate or discourage their children. Here the children are feeling that deep sense of frustration because their parents are not responding in an appropriate manner. Finally, there are many passages on God's wrath. In John 3, Jesus talked about those who reject him as those who had God's wrath resting on them.

In chapter 1 we examined Ephesians 4:26–27. Let's take two components of that verse and apply it to the Mountainview deacons meeting.

In your anger do not sin.

Garth was clearly angry. That is not a debatable point. He exploded in his anger and everyone in the room was aware of it. There is a sense in which Doreen was angry as well, but her anger was more implosive. She turned it on herself after she got home from the meeting. Was either of them sinning in their anger?

Remember we looked at the Greek word *thumos*—boiling, turbulent commotion. It is translated as "rage" or "fits

Sin or Righteousness?

of rage" in various passages of the New Testament. Because it reflects a complete lack of control, it is always linked with sin. Typically, rage is expressed without the best interests of the other in mind. In light of that, it falls short of the biblical standard of love and into the category of sin. In this case, the expression of Garth's anger was sinful.

What if Garth had responded differently? He would still be carrying a threatened sense of self-worth, but let's reconceptualize the meeting as follows:

"Garth, I think we need to go to the church and make sure we have broad ownership of this concept."

"Doreen, I think I understand the concept but I am not convinced we need to do that. Can you tell me more?"

"I'm not sure there is more to say. I just worry about making an independent decision without involving the whole community of faith."

"I disagree with what you are saying. I think we need to proceed on our own. Most in the church are trusting us to make these kinds of decisions. What do the rest of you think?"

Garth has clearly expressed his disagreement and has not gone into a rage. He has carried on a civil conversation. There is no overt indication of *thumos* anger. But, as has already been noted, the term "anger" in this verse is *orge*. This is the term that reflects an inner attitude or disposition that may lead to revenge or personal animosity. In our reconceptualized scenario above, we do not see any obvious revenge or animosity, but that could take place after the meeting. Garth could still go home and get into his "Doreen bashing" in his head.

Then there is Doreen. In the meeting she buckled to the power of Garth's anger and sacrificed what she believed to be important. After she got home she was frustrated with herself because this is a habitual response. Her anger is not with Garth, but with herself. Is her anger sin? Clearly the phrase "In your anger do not sin" is focused on our response to others, but the principles can be applied to what we have called implosive anger. Doreen's anger is more of the settled habit of the mind, or *orge* anger. She is sitting quietly in her condominium reflecting on the present and the past and confronting some important truths about herself. On the particular night in question, she is not experiencing personal animosity toward herself. The focus is more on being honest with herself and trying to deal with a powerful historical theme. In her anger she is not sinning.

Do not let the sun go down while you are still angry.

Early on Tuesday morning Garth is tossing and turning in bed and he is angry. He is compiling a list of Doreen's "sins" and his hostility is running deep. Eventually he falls asleep. We have already commented on the inaccurate rendering of this verse—Garth is not in sin because he fell asleep while he was still angry! The phrase indicates that the nurturing of anger over time may create irritation and exasperation, which eventually could lead to bitterness. The key question is not whether or not Garth fell asleep, but what he is going to do with his anger toward Doreen the next day. What did he do? After his interaction with Dorothy, he was able to understand what happened, got on the phone, and resolved the problem. By utilizing this strategy Garth did not only bring peace to a fractured relationship, he also did not "give the devil a foothold."

Doreen's situation is a little different, but the potential for nurturing anger over time so that it turns into bitterness is definitely there. Her anger at herself is linked with her father. In many ways she has a choice. She can live a life of frustration because of that relationship and even cultivate feelings of bitterness towards her dad, or she can continue to deal with the issues, either through personal

Sin or Righteousness?

work or with the help of a pastoral counselor. The way she handles it will probably have a large influence on whether or not the door is open for the devil.

It is extremely important to understand the process of resolving anger. It is not enough to come crashing into Garth's situation and say he is sinning and wrong and unbiblical. Over a short period of time, through his own reflection and his wife's insight, he was able to come to terms with what happened and move toward harmony and health. Our emphasis needs to be there. We need to acknowledge and accept our anger, determine whether it is something that God approves of, and then move to restoring fractured relationships.

Personal Reflections

1. Many of us spend time in small group meetings, like the deacons group under discussion in this chapter. It may be in the context of church, work, a social club, a community group, or whatever. Think back to a recent example of conflict in your group. Are there "Garths" in your group? "Doreens"? "Michaels"? Where do you fit, in terms of the way you handle anger in a meeting?
2. Garth and Doreen were able to gain insight when some time had passed after the meeting. Some people are like that by disposition. They do not fully understand what is going on around them or inside them at the time, but they can process it more accurately later. The key is that these people need to give themselves both permission and a space to do that. Are you like that? Do you intentionally allow yourself the freedom to do the processing after a meeting where there has been conflict?

3. Do you have a spouse, friend, or roommate that could function like Dorothy functioned with Garth? Can you ask them explicitly to help you talk through a difficult situation so your insight is deepened? Often our best self-understanding is cultivated in community.
4. Keep a journal of times when you are angry in the next week. Simply write down the feeling and the situation in which it occurred. When the week is over, go back to each situation and ask the why question: Why did I get angry in that situation? See how many incidents force you to look in at thwarted goals, values, expectations, or self-worth and how many put you into the blame game where you are holding someone else responsible. Make some decisions about how you would like to live in this particular area.
5. Garth became aware that his battered personal worth had played a major role in his display of anger. All of us have had difficult experiences in life where our personal worth becomes threatened, damaged, or bruised. How would you assess your sense of personal worth at the present time? Is any work needed in this sphere of life? Are you seeing any indications that you are responding to feedback or constructive criticism with defensiveness and fear?
6. The next time you are angry with someone for what they did or said or did not do or did not say, work through the Person (P) material that you brought to the event and then sit down with them and talk through it. Often in social interaction we are able to clarify some of our own baggage, and we also are letting the person know that they are not completely to blame for what went on.
7. Take out some paper and complete the following sentences: Feelings . . . ; God thinks that feelings . . . ; My family taught me that feelings . . . ; When I see

Sin or Righteousness?

people show their feelings I . . . ; When I think of feelings, I wish. . . . Answer honestly and openly by writing down the first thing that comes into your mind. When you have finished, do not reread it. A week later come back to what you have written and see what it tells you about yourself. What areas need work? How does your history with feelings affect the way you are at present?

8. Take the threefold distinction between acknowledge, accept, and approve and use it to analyze various feelings, including anger. Do you work through all these stages, or are you a person who quickly jumps to the conclusion "I should not be feeling that" before you have fully acknowledged and accepted that you are feeling it?

9. Read through the Gospels (Matthew, Mark, Luke, and John) and make a note of every passage that comments on or alludes to self-righteousness. Commit a few of the key passages to memory and pray that you will keep this mask out of your life.

10. In evangelical circles you will hear the phrase "righteous indignation" used when the topic of anger comes up. Unfortunately, this is a noncommunicative phrase in that everyone will have different criteria for the nature of "righteous" and "indignation." It is much more helpful to speak of some of the words used in Scripture. For example, *thumos* and *orge* provide us with three viewpoints on anger. In all cases, the fits of rage described in the first word are wrong. In the second word, we can be angry with or without a spirit of personal animosity and vengeance lurking behind it. Ask the Lord to give you clarity on the difference between these three and use them as a grid or paradigm to bring to the world of anger.

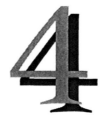

TRIGGERS AND THOUGHTS
THINKING EFFECTIVELY ABOUT YOUR ANGER

Summary: Garth decides to talk to his pastor to determine some of the key issues regarding his anger. He is unsure of why he is angry about the forced retirement and others are not. He is also unclear on what triggered inside of him. The importance of understanding the triggers is discussed and their rootedness in our personal history. Lurking behind those triggers are thought patterns that are resident in our goals, values, expectations, and personal worth. Approaching this with genuine humility and accuracy will help us coexist with others who do things differently than we do.

Self-Exploration in Community

It is now a few weeks after the deacons meeting and Garth has decided to go in to talk with his pastor. The focus for him is not on the meeting, but on some of the issues underlying it, particularly his anger. It has been some time since he was forced to retire, but he does not seem able to get a handle on the anger. He has come to a dead end in trying to figure it all out on his own so he thought it would be helpful to talk to someone else. While he has other friends that were let go, they do not seem to be having the same kinds of problems. And he still does not fully understand what triggered the problems in the meeting. He knows that Doreen tripped off something inside of him, but he is not quite clear what it is. He has a lot of respect for his pastor and believes that he may have some insights that will help in the process.

Only through self-exploration can we come to understand our own anger in its many dimensions. Only through having a safe context in which to explore and share with another is it possible for us to reveal and experience being understood by the other. It is interesting that self-exploration is seldom effective when entered into in isolation. One of the authors asked a colleague about a particular issue and was told, "I don't know. I haven't said it yet!" He went on to say that he often did not know what he thought about something until he had an interactive environment in which to explore the matter. Often, while our thoughts are rambling about in our gray matter, we are juggling so many bits and pieces that they don't seem to fit or correlate. However, in a nonjudgmental and accepting environment we may be encouraged to express these confused ramblings and in doing so we revise, adjust, elaborate, or affirm until a coherent pattern takes shape and we can say, "This is what I think." While Garth did not understand all the issues involved in self-exploration, he had an intuitive sense that he could not go the autonomous route.

Anger and the Body

Garth is wondering why his experience of anger is different from his former colleagues. Again, we come back to the uniqueness of anger, even in a physiological sense. Obviously, the organs, glands, muscles, and so on of the body function similarly in each of us, but there are differences as a result of genetics or experience. These differences may be subtle, but significant. If you have less propensity to gastrointestinal discomfort than someone else, you may be less conscious or less affected by the motility that comes as adrenaline is pumped into the stomach as part of the experience of anger.

You may recall in the first chapter that when Old Testament views of anger were discussed, it was noted that a number of the words for anger were associated with bodily functions. Anger locates itself or makes its presence felt in different parts of the body. However, we will vary in our consciousness of this. One person may say, "My heart is racing." Another may say, "My stomach is in knots." Another, "You make my head ache." All may be experiencing anger. It is helpful to get in touch with one's physiological experience of anger. That may, in fact, help us to identify anger when unconsciously we may be trying to mask it in other ways. Awareness of one's physiological response may be a first front of awareness in acknowledging and accepting anger.

There is a very close and synergistic relationship between our emotions and our body, especially with respect to anger and related emotions. For instance, Paul Brand (1993) writes about the dreaded condition known as reflex sympathetic dystrophy (RSD), a disorder that can render the hand completely stiff. He argues that simple fear or anger can produce this level of physical dysfunction in some people. There is no question that the general physiological response of the body to anger is personalized in the way we physically experience anger in our bodies. In this sense, anger is very personal and unique to each of us.

Permitting each other to have different experiences and different understandings of the same experience acknowledges the personal differences in anger. This requires that we explore and honor the differences. It is necessary that we, with humility, permit others to see and experience things differently than we do and not try to impose on others our experience or understanding. For Garth, this was a very important concern. He ran the risk of seeing others' responses as inappropriate or, as was his more current pattern, he could fall into the trap of being overly self-critical of his own reaction.

Unique Personal Triggers

Garth is also struggling with the link between the meeting and his anger. He knows there is some connection, but it is hard to figure out precisely what triggered his reaction. Have you noticed how often our anger is activated by essentially insignificant happenings? Why would anyone go berserk and bang a table over the congregation making a decision about a parking lot expansion? But it happens to all of us and it is really confusing. Some little thing sets us off! It may be a look, a gesture, or a thoughtless act. We are gone, into orbit and out of control. And, of course, our response may be as confusing to us as it is to those who witness it.

There are a variety of analogies that may help us to understand what is happening here. We may look at the stimulus that activates us as a trigger. When firing a rifle the very slight pull on the trigger activates a mechanism called the firing pin, which is housed in a bolt. The firing pin impacts a primer resulting in a very small spark within the primer. That small spark exits into a chamber which con-

Thinking Effectively about Your Anger

tains very explosive material, which when ignited creates extreme pressure, which pushes the bullet down the barrel into the outside world. The devastating impact of the bullet is far-reaching compared to the insignificant movement of the trigger.

The question "What lights your fuse?" raises another analogy to explain triggers. The fuse may be ignited by a very small flame. The fuse may be short or long, which determines the time lapse between the lighting of the fuse and the explosion of the "bomb" at the other end. Sometimes there is a delay between the igniting of the fuse and the explosion. So it is with anger. It only takes a small spark to get an explosion activated.

Each of us will have different triggers. This is one of the major spheres in which the personal side of anger manifests itself. Different things light our fuses. Exploring these triggers will help us to understand what sets us off. A willingness to see that others have different triggers and opening ourselves to explore and honor the triggers of others may lead to much learning. Mountainview Bible Church, like any church, had many triggers to set off anger. The trigger for Sally was that other woman raising her hands. For Helmut, it was the memory of Bonnie's stubborn rejection of his advances. Elisabeth's fuse was lit by the attention Doreen drew to herself. Tom was fired up by a breach of his preferences. And Garth? A rather insignificant, at least to Doreen, suggestion about communal decision making became a powerful stimulus for anger.

Cataloguing your triggers requires that you take the focus off the expression of anger, and focus on understanding the context in which you experience the stimulus. We can only guess at what was triggered in the people in the church. At a very superficial level, the waving hands may simply have been blocking Sally's view. Could it be, at another level, that she would like to be more expressive in worship? Or, could it be that she has felt "blocked" as a more general experience of life? Being the youngest child, smaller than all her siblings, she felt lost in the world of kneecaps while she grew up. Her view may have literally been blocked. Perhaps her expression of herself was blocked. It may be that early marriage blocked her fulfillment of vocational dreams. If we explored with Sally what it means to be blocked or distracted or inhibited, would we come to understand her trigger that activated her anger that morning in church?

What was the trigger for Doreen? She chatted with one of her friends about the infamous meeting, and after a lengthy conversation her friend asked her to use an image or analogy to describe what she felt when she got home after the meeting. Immediately Doreen, who had been relaying the incident quite calmly, broke into uncontrollable sobs. Through her tears she blurted out, "I felt boxed in." Then out came an emotionally laden experience from her history. She went back to her childhood experience of playing with older siblings who on occasion put her in a box, closed the lid, and then ran away to hide. She was not strong enough to get out of the box, panicked, and became fearful and angry. The control she was experiencing from a rather rigid, somewhat autocratic chair of the deacons triggered feelings of smallness, of being overpowered and not being heard, as well as the danger of being rejected if she didn't cooperate. The trigger in the present activated feelings, thoughts, and even physical sensations that were not at all at the level of her consciousness. Frequently, we may get in touch with the fact that triggers may be activating deeply embedded fears or patterns of thought that have little to do with the present.

In interaction with the pastor, Garth also became aware of some historical problems that were triggered by the meeting. There was the immediate situation of being replaced by a younger woman at his job. Although he did not know her, he found that he resented this inexperienced woman replacing him after he had devoted his life to work. It was that latter phrase that the pastor picked up on.

"In what sense did you devote your life to work?"

"Life was my work. I loved what I did. It was where I felt most comfortable. I had been there for thirty-one years. I felt like they wanted me and I needed them. And it was my first full-time job. I started there when I was twenty-six."

Garth goes on to relay the scenario that occurred when he was twenty-six. He had gone to university when he was twenty and had obtained a general science degree there. Then he took two years off to save enough money for medical school. He worked long and hard hours and eventually when we was twenty-five he started pursuing his medical degree. Two weeks into his program his parents were both killed in a car accident. It was a whirlwind few weeks. He had to take care of his younger siblings who were all living at home, which meant he had to take time off from school. Then he found out that his parents had almost no life insurance, so he had to take a job that paid well but was outside of his interests in science and medicine. He had very little time to process all that had happened, but he poured himself into his job so he could be the provider for his brothers and sisters. Not long after that, he met Dorothy and they got married following a brief courtship. The marriage has been tolerable, but not terribly stimulating. Slowly he moved more heavily into work responsibilities so he would not have to deal with the grief issues from his parents' deaths or his inner sense of marital dissatisfaction. He felt disconnected from people and from himself, but work gave him a place of connection and belonging. The conflict of the deacons meeting triggered a number of these themes and made him angry.

The sensations we experience associated with the triggers of anger are important keys to unlocking the mystery of anger. Often we do not rationally understand, nor do others, why we respond with the reaction we do. The sensation of being boxed, suffocated, pressured, pressed on all sides, being between a rock and a hard place, being on slippery footing, or any other sensation that is associated with our anger may often help in exploring it. Again, it is a matter of taking the feeling seriously and seeking in the context of a relationship to not just understand the stimulus in the environment but the trigger inside of us.

This strategy requires that we "stay with" the anger. Sometimes when we are angry we react to our reaction. Do you remember Judith who was sitting in the service still struggling with her anger at her kids? She had gone in to her nine year old's room that morning and found him writing with nonerasable marker all over the walls, the walls that she had just painted last month. She was very angry with him, partially because of what he was doing to the walls, but more at the fact that as a nine year old he was fully aware that this was not appropriate behavior. But in church she was not processing her anger and seeking to understand the trigger. She was exasperated with herself because she got angry. What that did was add another layer on. She had the original anger to deal with, but was now plagued with a sense of exasperation combined with guilt. It was this second layer that became her focus of attention. In contrast, if she had "stayed with" her original anger, she would have realized that an angry response to her child's destructive behavior is probably appropriate.

Thinking Clearly When Angry

Thinking clearly when angry sounds like an oxymoron. It is certain that most of us feel we do not do our clearest thinking when angry. On the other hand, if we are to understand anger, we must learn to think about our experience of it differently and learn to think about finding alternative and more effective ways to express it.

If we come to understand what our triggers are, we have made a start to thinking differently. Seeing the immediate provocation to anger as only a trigger, which activates something deeper, suggests that we must look beyond the immediate trigger of our anger to find and understand its true source. But we need to understand the thinking that lurks behind the trigger. Three examples will illustrate this.

For Doreen, her anger at herself was triggered by Garth's anger. Her feeling was that of being boxed in. In the recesses of her memory, she had feelings and thoughts related to childhood experiences. She thought of herself as small, powerless, and rejected by older siblings. Going behind the trigger would necessitate exploring, acknowledging, and coming to grips with those feelings, which had become part of her image of herself.

The children of Israel sent spies into the Promised Land at God's suggestion. Ten of the twelve spies (Num. 13) gave an evil report to the children of Israel. Their report concerning the produce, the cities, and the people was accurate and truthful. The evil was expressed in the last sentence of their report: "We seemed like grasshoppers in our own eyes, and we looked the same to them" (13:33). What the children of Israel thought about themselves determined their response. A "grasshopper perspective" of one's self provides the foundation for responding with flight from a threatening experience. The trigger was the Nephilim, but the real problem was the way the Israelites thought of themselves. They created an additional problem by projecting the image that they had of themselves onto the Nephilim and assuming that the Nephilim thought similarly of them. This was a lie. There is no evidence that their attitude toward the children of Israel was such. God's people turned away to wander in the wilderness, turning their backs upon the victory God was about to give them and rebelling in their stubbornness.

Jonah had a problem with anger. The Bible says, "Jonah was greatly displeased and became angry" (Jonah 4:1). He felt so good about his anger that he went immediately to prayer to complain not only *to* God, but *about* God. That must have taken a considerable amount of pride in his own rightness of perspective. He wasn't even tentative about his accusation against God! He was so offended and angry that he wanted to die, as he said, "I am angry enough to die" (4:9). What was his problem? He thought very differently about the Ninevites than God did. He knew God was gracious, compassionate, and abounding in love toward them, but he thought differently.

In these three illustrations, we see problems in thinking. Doreen's thinking, which was shaped by thoughts, feelings, and attitudes related to her childhood, determined her response to Garth who provided a trigger to activate that response. She was not fully aware of the relationship between her response to Garth and the experiences of childhood until she talked with a friend. The children of Israel consciously thought of themselves as grasshoppers in comparison to the Nephilim and then projected that self-perception on the Nephilim and responded as if it were true. Jonah thought of the Ninevites very differently than God did. His values and expectations were very different from God's, in spite of the fact that he knew God and could articulate his qualities. The arrogance of his pride was profound.

Let's return to Garth. He talked to the pastor because he did not know why others were not obsessed with the downsizing and forced retirement and he could not fully understand the link between his history and his response in the meeting. As we have already seen, one of the major dynamics of anger is that it is personal and individual, particularly around physiological issues. No two people are going to respond exactly alike. But there is also a uniqueness in the triggers. Garth's history has been pulled out in the present. He is emotionally responding to a present cir-

Thinking Effectively about Your Anger

cumstance from the context of his whole life. But what about Garth's thoughts? What is he thinking? Like Doreen, the children of Israel, and Jonah, Garth has thoughts that are playing a role.

This perspective moves us into a very important area of Scripture. Fundamentally, our mind or inner attitude needs to be focused on the injunction of Philippians 2:5: "Your attitude should be the same as that of Christ Jesus." We are to seek to bring our minds to think about things in certain ways. We are to seek as believers to come to a sameness of mind as we follow Christ (Rom. 12:16; 15:5; Phil. 2:2). This will affect the way we view things (Gal. 5:10). The word is used in the way we would ask someone for their views concerning something (Acts 28:22), or the way we feel (Phil. 1:7) or care about someone (Phil. 4:10). It is a serious word, describing the non-Christians who have "their minds set" on the sinful nature (Rom. 8:5).

In Romans (12:3, 16) we read, "Do not think of yourself more highly than you ought, but rather think of yourself with sober judgment, in accordance with the measure of faith God has given you. . . . do not be proud." There is a prideful way to think. The alternative is to think of one's self with "sober judgment." The term "sober judgment" is probably best translated as "accurate." In other words, think of yourself accurately. This is the opposite of pride, where there is an overinflated view of self. Humility, in contrast, gives us a more balanced and reality-based view of self that is reflected in our thinking. Such is the description of the man Jesus rescued from the demons who is described as "in his right mind" (Mark 5:15). Paul urges young men to be self-controlled or discreet (Titus 2:6). Peter urges us to "be clear minded and self-controlled so that you can pray" (1 Peter 4:7).

How ought we to think? Paul tells us that, "When I was a child, I talked like a child, I thought like a child, I reasoned like a child. When I became a man, I put childish ways behind me" (1 Cor. 13:11). When we bring energy from our childhood, which implodes or explodes in response to triggers in the present, it may be that we are talking, thinking, and reasoning out of that childhood pain. Often we will be unconscious of that fact. It takes courage to explore it, to acknowledge it, to own it, and to free ourselves so we are not enslaved to that past. Only by freeing ourselves from the past can we understand the present with accuracy and respond to it with honesty. The battle for this will be largely fought in the mind.

Freedom in Humility

The humility of mind mentioned in Philippians 2:3 is demonstrated by Christ Jesus as Paul presents him in verses 5 through 11. He focused on the "interests of others" (v. 4) by "doing nothing out of selfish ambition or vain conceit" (v. 3). The orientation of his thinking was the interest of others. His reaction to others was to focus his attention on their interests. His mental attitude toward himself was to empty himself, taking the form of a servant, humbling himself to become obedient even to the extreme of death for others.

How do we achieve this attitude of mind? To begin, we can only be free from the defensiveness that arises out of our captivity to the pain of our past by pursuing healing from those pains. If we are unaware of the pains of the past or the patterns that are the fruit on our family trees, we will always function with the pain or pattern of those experiences. You can imagine having a conversation with Michael about these things. It might go something like this.

"I don't understand all this history talk. The past is gone and we should get on with our lives and live the way God wants us to. I don't struggle with anger from my past and I don't have any problems with it now. I find it very sad when I see situations like the one with Garth. If he could just get beyond his past he would be all right."

Michael expresses a sentiment that is not that atypical in Christian circles: Forget the past and get on with your life. The irony is that people who have an understanding of their past and are willing to deal with the themes and patterns that come out of it are open to experience much more healing and growth. In fact, they are no longer victimized by their past because they have been able to identify significant patterns that they are open to processing. In contrast, someone like Michael is out of touch with the effect of his own history, which makes him a victim of it. The deacons meeting is a good example. He thought he was doing the right and Christian thing by shutting off the feelings of Garth and Doreen. The reality is that he did this because he was living out of the patchwork of his own family background. In a sense, he was a victim of his own history but did not know it.

Humility both frees us from the tyranny of self and gives us a mind-set that acknowledges our dependence upon, and enabling by, God's Spirit. Thus, we enter the adventure of dealing with our struggles with a clear anticipation of victory. Being free from self, we can be free for others. We can open ourselves to their perspective with empathy and understanding. Grace frees us from the tyranny of shame, guilt, or blame so that we can stand tall in God's grace as we seek to follow the model of Christ Jesus.

We can only overcome a "grasshopper perspective" by seeing ourselves from God's grace perspective. A grace perspective sees one's self as being indwelt, ministered to, and enabled by the Spirit. It is his grace that has distributed the gifts in the body. It is his grace that has given us our identity. That is why Paul could say, "By the grace of God I am what I am" (1 Cor. 15:10) or "I can do everything through him who gives me strength" (Phil. 4:13). This is precisely where Jonah got into trouble with his anger. In contrast to the mind of Christ, Jonah could not tolerate God being compassionate toward someone to whom he felt no compassion. He did not have the mind of God, even though he knew the character of God. The truth is that knowledge does not always lead to the right behavior. We must bring our values and expectations into line with those of God.

Dissecting the Thinking

Imagine being confronted by Sally after the Mountainview Bible Church morning service. She says to you what she said to William: "Could you believe that woman with her hands in the air during the singing this morning? How could you miss that obvious display of self-centeredness?" William did not see the woman and Sally left him more frustrated than when she first came up to him. To this point in the chapter we have learned that there are different physiological reactions to given stimuli. Would you have reacted the way Sally responded? We have also learned that there are unique triggers that are usually resident in our family history. Do you have any historical issues that would have elicited anger in this situation?

We talked earlier about goals, values, expectations, and personal worth. Let's reformulate those in thinking language. As we talk about Sally, go through the process for yourself. What is a goal? A goal is something that I am striving for. What is the source of that goal? My thinking. Let's say Sally has come to church with the unconscious thought going through her head, "I want this service to make me happy." Her goal is to make sure that the service brings that kind of personal contentment. She wants to leave happy. When the hands go in the air, she is not happy and is therefore angry. Why is she angry? Notice, the anger is not there because there are hands in the air. She is angry because her goal has been thwarted. But it goes deeper than that.

Thinking Effectively about Your Anger

What is a value? A value is a core belief, something that I cherish and prize. It is a standard that is resident in my thinking and one that is held in high esteem. Maybe Sally values reflective and pensive worship. She likes things to be calm in worship. She loves that verse that says things at church should be done "decently and in order." She is not quite sure what that means or even where it is found in the New Testament, but for her it means you are not demonstrative in worship, especially physically. Worship is about the mind, not the body. Why is she angry? Not because the hands are in the air, but because one of her values has been blocked.

What is an expectation? It is a belief about what is proper and necessary. In our thinking we all have beliefs about the way others should be. Often it is a move from simply having a value to believing that other people should hold the same value. In fact, if we experience a lot of anger, much of it ties in with the fact that other people are not doing what we believe they should be doing. In this case, Sally has a value about expressive worship, which in turn is linked with an expectation. If she believes raising hands is not an appropriate response in worship, then others should not be doing it. Why is she angry? Hands in the air do not precipitate anger, but broken expectations do.

What is personal worth? It is my sense of well-being, my identity, the degree to which I am comfortable with who I am and what I believe. In Sally's case, her self-worth is very much tied to others agreeing with and validating her beliefs. For her, differences are wrong and bad. They cannot be tolerated. If you do not agree with her, then that makes her a less-than-good person. It makes her feel insecure and that is overwhelming for her. In order to preserve who she is, it is very important that everyone be on the same page. Why is she angry? Not because of expressive worship, but because she is feeling personally threatened.

Notice that the content of these various areas is not feeling based but thinking oriented:

Goal: I want to be happy.
Value: Reflective and pensive worship is right.
Expectation: Others should not engage in expressive worship.
Personal worth: I am a good person if others agree with me.

Something as simple as someone putting their hands in the air violates Sally's goal, value, expectation, and personal worth. As others interact with her, they may be tempted to say she is getting upset over nothing, but these thoughts are deeply embedded in her and will not simply cease because others question their validity. What she needs is an infusion of humility through the work of the Holy Spirit and the mediation of the body of Christ. We are not being simplistic in saying this, but the arrogance of Sally's thinking, in a nonbiblical area, will only be softened when she comes to terms with the superiority that is embedded in it. Styles of worship are a personal issue that can be traced to theological, personal, and denominational history. Sally is not the ultimate authority on which style is most acceptable.

Note the substantial difference if Sally's thoughts were to shift to the following:

Goal: I want everyone in a worship service to express themselves with integrity.
Value: I value diversity in the body of Christ, so difference is neither right nor wrong.
Expectation: I do not expect anyone else to be exactly like me.
Personal worth: My value is not dependent on what others do or do not do.

There is more humility in these thoughts and they are more consistent with biblical standards. If Sally brought this mind-set to church, she would experience very little anger.

But What about the Other Person?

At this point, you may be feeling the focus is too much on our experience of anger and not enough on the person provoking the anger. After all, we do need to look at this trigger and the person who is providing that stimulus. This is true. However, it is important to take responsibility for ourselves and to have the courage and humility for self-exploration. Out of our understanding of ourselves, we can take responsibility for our own actions, responses, and the outcomes in our lives. After all, it is our anger we are seeking to deal with.

We do need to look at the person or situation that provides the trigger, but it is important that we have the mind-set that will enable us to see what is truly there rather than a distortion or projection. The children of Israel projected a perception onto the Nephilim that was not what the Nephilim thought at all. Jonah projected a value onto the Ninevites that did not correspond to God's value of them. It is helpful if we become very cautious and tentative in projecting onto others perceptions, attitudes, motives, or intentions that are, in fact, only our guess. The attribution of intent to another is a guessing game. It is a bit like gambling. The odds that we will guess right are very much stacked against us.

Attribution intention to another person may express arrogance and pride. It is based upon the assumption that my perspective is right or accurate, or perhaps that my perspective is the only one or the correct one. It is not quite so easy to enter another's being and to see the world through their eyes and to understand experience through their mind. The way of humility is to withhold judgment and to seek openly to explore and understand the other's perspective or intention. To do that we have to withhold judgment, assessment, criticism, evaluation, diagnosis, or verdict until we have explored and understood the other person. This is really difficult.

We are trained from babyhood to differentiate, distinguish, and enter into many forms of evaluation. It becomes second nature. We leap to such mental assessment or attribution of intention and meaning to another's behavior. That is really what caused Garth so much difficulty when he got home from the meeting. Apart from what actually happened, he had to deal with what he was imagining as well. His mind-set needed to shift from this style to a pattern that withholds judgment. He also needed to be open to an exploration of Doreen's meaning or intention.

To do these things well, we need a magnanimous spirit that is generous and accepting. This is exactly what Paul urges us to in Philippians 4:5: "Let your gentleness be evident to all." The word "gentleness" could be translated "magnanimous, generous, or reasonable." Such an attitude or mind-set would open us to the second step, which is to explore the meaning or intention of the other person. If Garth could have withheld his attribution of intention and opened himself to explore Doreen's meaning, he probably would have been able to sleep much earlier. Usually, when we respond with a knee-jerk response or from an autopilot reflex action, we misrepresent the person's intent. In addition, we are usually responding out of an unnecessarily defensive or protective posture.

In order to accomplish this change in response pattern, we must clearly plan it in our minds before we experience the stimulation of the moment. Trouble comes when we respond with an autopilot response, which is determined by previous experience rather than assessing the present through openness and interaction. It is our reflex responses that are learned by the conditioning of the past. Change of thinking occurs when we prethink situations before we experience them. To state this as a principle, we must clarify our commitments prior to the test of circumstances. If we want to change our responses to a given stimulus, we must preplan a different response and have that new response so clearly fixed in our minds that when the stimulus occurs we will respond in a new way. Thus, we free ourselves from old patterns of thought and develop more helpful and effective ways of thinking and responding.

So after his interaction with the pastor, Garth might realize that his sense of personal worth and identity is threatened when he is in a situation with younger females. Recognizing that, he could plan a different kind of response when he feels the emotion of anger being triggered. Rather than letting the other person have it, he could take more ownership for the problem and not dump it on others. Notice, this approach does not cure his anger problem, but helps position it in the proper sphere for ongoing resolution.

In discussing the imputation of good intention, we are aware that this is not always the case. Not everyone has good intentions or motives toward us. There is evil in the world. However, in most cases we are dealing with people who love us or care for us or, at minimum, are not out to get us. Their intentions are good. In fact, often when we have exploded toward another person they say, "But that was not what I meant or intended." We have all experienced the guilt or shame of attributing to someone intention that we later discover was not accurate.

At times people do not clearly express their intention. Maybe they have garbled the message. If this is so, then our response of exploration and the pursuit of understanding will give them an accepting context to correct or clarify what their intention really was. Even if they garbled the message, we do not benefit from imploding or exploding in ways that are to our own detriment. It is better to clarify the message than to respond in self-harming ways to a garbled message.

If we can approach the situation with a mind-set that will enable us to think differently about anger, we have the potential to unscramble the message and to respond to the real intent or meaning of the person. If we discover that our anger is evoked by a breach of goals, values, expectations, or our sense of worth, we can respond out of that awareness. We can then check that out with the person involved. We can talk about whether we do, in fact, have a difference in the goals, values, or expectations that are at issue. And we can raise the question as to whether it was their intent to devalue us and breach our sense of worth. Rationally discussing the situation will be a better alternative than entering into the behavior of anger which we, very likely, both fear and which can be so destructive.

In discovering a more effective way to think about our anger, we have new tools with which to explore and to articulate what is of concern to us. If the other person will make a similar commitment, we have the best possibility for the experience of understanding. If the other person does not wish or is unable to enter into this process, we still have the benefit of our own self-understanding and a more effective means of expressing ourselves than the destructive process of imploding or exploding.

Personal Reflections

1. Garth made a decision to do his self-exploration in the context of community; that is, he decided to seek out the help of his pastor to provide insight and perspective. Outside help can be personal from a friend, pastoral from someone in that role, or professional from a trained counselor. As you reflect on your own anger issues, list a couple of people who might fit

into each of these categories. Are you at a stage where you would benefit from some outside help?
2. Given the link of anger with the body, do an inventory on yourself. The next time you are angry, tune in to your body. What are you feeling? Where are you feeling it? What kinds of sensations are going through your body? Do you get sick or have unusual aches or pains when you are intensely angry? This level of self-awareness can often make us more conscious of when we are angry and why.
3. We have talked about rifles and fuses to illustrate triggers. Can you think of other images or symbols that represent triggers? How do these images help you understand your own anger?
4. Let us suggest that you explore your triggers. One way to do this is to explore your feelings at the triggering point in the equation of anger. Find an analogy, a picture of how you felt at that point. Would the word "blocked," "frustrated," "steamed," "exasperated," "put down," "overlooked," "run over," "stabbed," or "forgotten" best describe your sensation at that point? You add your words. Creating imagery that captures and pictures your feelings or thoughts related to the triggering of anger is very helpful. The imagery you create may enable self-exploration.
5. We have provided brief biographical sketches of Garth, Doreen, and Sally. Do a brief sketch of yourself by noting a few key incidents that you think have produced triggers. This is not a form of a "blame game" in that we are trying to get you to dump on your past. It is more for the benefit of fresh understanding so that you can take full responsibility for your reactions.
6. Read the fourth chapter of Jonah carefully. Picture what happened in your mind. Obviously, the chapter does not outline all the details, but see if you can fill some in. What do you think Jonah was going

through? What was he feeling? What kinds of physiological responses were present? Can you put some specific sentences under Jonah's goals, values, expectations, and personal worth? What was God going through as he listened to Jonah? Explore this entire story in some depth and detail.

7. Philippians 2:5 is an extremely important verse to understand. What does it mean to you? How can you put it into practice specifically? Do a study of the verse by linking other relevant passages with it.

8. "Pride" and "humility" are two of those words that we hear and think we understand but there is a lot more to them than we realize. Take two sheets of paper. At the top of one of them write: Times When I Am Humble; at the top of the other: Times When I Am Proud. Obviously, the first sheet runs some risks, but you are not bragging about your humility—just trying to understand how it shows itself in your life! Do you have any examples that tie into any of our discussions on these topics?

9. The next time you are angry at something or someone, write one sentence beside goal, value, expectation, and personal worth. Write specific and succinct sentences that capture the thinking process you were going through at the time of anger. Then write four other sentences that would not have produced anger. Make some decisions to clarify your commitments before you hit particular circumstances.

10. As people respond toward you, become conscious of the distinction between behavior and intention. On the one hand, this is what they are doing. On the other, this is what they intend. Watch and see whether you attribute intent to others' behavior and what happens to you when you do. In close relationships, watch the natural tendency to get into conflict over what was meant, rather than what was done.

5

AVOIDING VENGEANCE
BEHAVING RIGHTEOUSLY

> Summary: A rather nasty confrontation occurs in the lobby of Mountainview Bible Church. This incident forms the backdrop for a discussion about the behavioral manifestations of anger. Because vengeance is a natural response when we are angry, we need to understand its dynamics carefully. Linked with this is the theme of forgiveness, a major antidote to anger. Finally, passive, aggressive, and assertive styles of communication allow us to express our anger in different ways.

The "Sharing Concerns" Syndrome

It is Sunday at 12:05 P.M. and we are back at Mountainview Bible Church. Bert has just finished teaching his Sunday school class and he is spent! He has a class of seven twelve-year-old boys and they push him to the limit. It is not that they are poorly behaved. On the whole they listen quite well and there is not too much conflict between them—but it's those questions! Every week they come up with more and more difficult questions and he wonders if he will ever be able to keep up with their inquisitive minds. Today was no different. He was talking about sin from Romans 1, but they were most interested in verse 20 and what it meant that humanity was without excuse because God had revealed himself in creation. They came at it from every angle, and on many of the issues Bert was stumped. But for him this was where the excitement in teaching came in. He liked it when the boys explored issues and thought through them for themselves.

He had just made his way around the corner into the front foyer when he was accosted by Salvatore. Accosted is the right word. Salvatore was fit to be tied. Bert could see it on his face before he opened his mouth.

"I want to share a concern with you. Could you tell me what on earth you are teaching my son in Sunday school? He comes home and he does not know up from down anymore. We have provided him with a good solid grounding in Scripture and I get the impression that you are undoing it systematically. I am going to talk to the Christian Education director about this and I really have serious questions about whether you should even be teaching. How are they going to move into the teenage years with this kind of wishy-washy approach to things? Do you come from a Christian background?"

Bert was lost for words. He knew that "sharing a concern" in some evangelical circles is a synonym for giving someone an angry blast, but he felt bombarded not just by Salvatore's words, but by the intensity, the hostility, and the raw emotion. He had enough sense to know that

Salvatore was not asking any questions, even though some of them were phrased that way, so he just waited and assumed that he would continue. It was an accurate assumption.

"Someone told me that you have some funny ideas about creation and that your positions are not always evangelical. That really concerns me. I want my son to grow up to know what he believes and why. I do not want the waters to get muddy simply because you do not know what you believe."

The Dynamics of Vengeance

In previous chapters we looked at one of the sinful manifestations of anger, namely, personal animosity and vengeance. One of the major ways these reactions are displayed is in behavior. The interaction between Bert and Salvatore illustrates this well. There is obvious anger, but at this point we are not sure exactly what triggered him or why he chose this moment to bombard Bert. His behavior has a vengeful tone to it, and there is a fair degree of personal animosity expressed covertly and overtly.

Let's focus our attention on a key passage of Scripture that helps us understand the dynamics of vengeance:

> Do not repay anyone evil for evil. Be careful to do what is right in the eyes of everybody. If it is possible, as far as it depends on you, live at peace with everyone. Do not take revenge, my friends, but leave room for God's wrath, for it is written: "It is mine to avenge; I will repay," says the Lord. On the contrary: "If your enemy is hungry, feed him; if he is thirsty, give him something to drink. In doing this, you will heap burning coals on his head." Do not be overcome by evil, but overcome evil with good. (Rom. 12:17–21)

The first sentence in this passage makes it clear that the natural tendency to repay evil for evil should not occur in any interpersonal situation. (This is in contrast to the governmental and civil sphere where authorities become "God's servants . . . agents of wrath" [13:4].) How does this happen? By "being careful to do what is right in the eyes of everybody." At first glance this seems like an invitation to be a people pleaser, to make sure everyone sees what you are doing. But Paul is arguing for planning ahead. When you are careful to do what is right, you are anticipating situations where difficulties may occur and deciding, in advance, that you will do the right thing. It is the same idea we have explored before. Settle your convictions before you hit particular circumstances. Then others will experience and observe your righteous behavior.

But this is not a guarantee that all relationships will work out well. There will be people who treat us poorly even though we are seeking to do what is right. Verse 18 captures this scenario. The sense of "if it is possible, as far as it depends on you" is that we need to do everything we can to be on proper terms with others. We need to exhaust all avenues in order to be at peace with others. However, this strategy does not necessarily lead to a positive outcome. Who is responsible for peace in a relationship? Both parties. Christians cannot make it their goal to be at peace with everyone, but it is their responsibility to "make every effort to live in peace with all" (Heb. 12:14).

This truth can be tremendously reassuring to people who feel guilty when relationships are not perfect. At times you can go to someone who is struggling with you and ask for forgiveness, request dialogue, or express a willingness to resolve the problems. In so doing, you are attempting to do all that you can to facilitate peace. You soon realize that not everyone is willing to pursue the avenue of peace. In those cases, your desire for resolution is not met with a mutual response. Reassurance can only come from the realization that you have made every effort.

Paul then returns in verse 19 to the absolute prohibition regarding vengeance by providing the rationale. Why should we not engage in "pay back" when someone wrongs us? Vengeance belongs to God. It is his prerogative and his responsibility. Since only God can judge human thought and intent with accuracy, he is much better equipped to respond to the evil that others do toward us. For us to take it on ourselves is to rob God of something that he owns: "It is mine to avenge; I will repay." So what is the alternative? Paul addresses this question in verse 20: "On the contrary."

While the Christian is not to even the score with the enemy, he or she is to reach out and minister. If they are hungry, they are to be given food. Drink is to be provided if they are thirsty. The enemy is not responded to in ways that correspond with their evil, but is cared for in terms of their own personal needs. The offended party does not make the enemy responsible horizontally, but commits them to God who will deal with their sin in his own way and time. In a similar fashion the offended party also becomes accountable to God by ministering to the enemy and giving them what they do not deserve.

This passage provides details on what it means to love others. Jesus had taught the importance of loving your enemies (Matt. 5:44), and Paul now demonstrates that this love is not an emotive response toward the other. Who feels positive toward those who are enemies? If anything, our enemies elicit negative feelings and hostile emotions. But the command to love is oriented more toward our knowledge and our will than our feelings. It is a command that addresses a behavioral ethic—feed him, give him something to drink. In doing this "you will heap burning coals on his head." At first glance, this may seem like a not-so-subtle form of vengeance. Respond to your enemy's needs and you will be able to get him back with burning coals. Obviously, this is not the thrust of the passage given what has preceded it. There are at least two other potential explanations. In its cultural setting, a pan of coals placed on the head was a public expression of repentance. Explicit deeds of kindness may provoke remorse. On the other hand, if your neighbor's fireplace had gone out, you could bring a burning coal to relight the flame, and in so doing express Christian charity. Behavioral expressions of love could result in either repentance or an experience of kindness.

Verse 21 of this chapter summarizes the argument succinctly. The presence of evil in interpersonal relationships allows for one of two responses—evil or good. The former is the route of vengeance, of evening the score or seeking personal justice. The latter is the path of love, of doing good and expressing kindness. This choice is difficult, as the term "overcome" reflects, a term that gives a sense of battle and conquering. But the bottom line is clear. We are not responsible for others' evil toward us, but we are responsible for our response to the evil.

How does Salvatore stack up against this passage? First, we do not know whether Bert was teaching heresy or not. It would appear that Bert's approach to teaching was more student directed and interactive, whereas Salvatore was looking for a more content centered, "tell it like it is" approach. They are probably in an extrabiblical realm rather than one that relates to truth or doctrine. But let's assume that Bert was teaching heresy. Is Salvatore's response appropriate? The timing was poor, his anger was out of control, and he gave the impression that he had personal animosity toward a fellow Christian. For Salvatore, Bert was "systematically" undermining the parental teaching on Scripture. He should probably not be teaching Sunday school and his approach is basically "wishy-washy." At the end Salvatore is even raising questions about whether he comes from a Christian background. Furthermore, he accuses Bert of having funny, nonevangelical views about creation and thinks that things are muddy because Bert does not know what he believes. Clearly Salvatore's response is vengeful and requires forgiveness.

Forgiveness and Vengeance

Later, in the parking lot, Bert is getting into his car and sees Salvatore coming in his direction. After the other incident he is braced for what might happen, but he is a little startled when Salvatore puts his arm around him and says, "I really lost it in there. Sorry about that. Forgive and forget?" Not knowing what else to do, Bert says, "Yeah. Sure. No problem."

What does it mean to forgive? Does forgiving mean forgetting? Does anger remain after forgiveness? David Augsburger (1984) talks about three important ingredients in forgiveness. The first is understanding the other person. When we are angry with someone we not only feel like expressing vengeance, but we are also short on understanding. In fact, we believe that the other person does not deserve our understanding. One aspect of forgiveness is the ability and the willingness to be understanding of the other person's experience. In doing this we are not trying to totally understand the other person and dissect all their motives and intents. Rather, we are seeking to recognize that there are reasons behind all of our actions and that all of us are not totally made up of negative qualities and actions. So when someone does something that upsets us, we recognize that there may have been reasons for this and, furthermore, there is more to this person than this one behavior.

Avoiding Vengeance

How does that apply in this situation? Does Bert understand Salvatore's experience? Does he know what was going on for him? Not at all. Their parking lot exchange makes it very difficult to know what he was thinking. In a sense, he is simply trying to cover it up. And let us turn it around from the other perspective. Salvatore has asked Bert to forgive him, but what about the reverse? Has Salvatore found out more information since the conversation so he genuinely understands what Bert is going through as a Sunday school teacher? Is it possible that he is simply requesting forgiveness in his own direction, but not willing to reciprocate?

The second component of forgiveness is valuing others. A logical extension of seeking to understand others is an ability to value and respect them. As people created in the image of God, and in our case redeemed by Jesus Christ, we are those that need to offer each other the gift of value. In this sense, no one is unlovable or undeserving of our forgiveness and compassion. In this situation, the interaction does not allow for a valuing of the other, in either direction. Minimal communication occurs so valuing the other is more of an abstract concept rather than a practical reality.

Augsburger's third point ties nicely into our discussion on Romans 12. He suggests that the third component of forgiveness is loving the other person. This quality is not something we can manufacture, but it is a gift from God. It is the divine power that allows us to feed our enemy when he is hungry, or give her a drink when she is thirsty. As we serve, help, give, and minister to others we become continually strengthened to complete the work of forgiveness in the sense that we are not holding things against others. Again, the brief exchange makes this an impossibility. More time and substance would be needed to bring this to fruition.

Luke 17:3–4 makes a startling statement about forgiveness: "If your brother sins, rebuke him, and if he repents, forgive him. If he sins against you seven times in a day, and seven times comes back to you and says, 'I repent,' forgive him." In this passage, forgiveness seems to be something that we are responsible to give others, quite apart from what they have done to us. We often think you can only forgive someone if they have repented genuinely. The individual in Luke 17 comes back after sinning seven times in one day and says, "I repent." There is no way that the person could have been genuine. Otherwise, they would not have kept sinning. But Jesus still says we are to forgive.

In response to this injunction, it is no wonder that the disciples asked the Lord to increase their faith. You would need a lot of faith to live that way. But Jesus contradicts that by talking about faith as a mustard seed and how we do not need much faith. Then later in the chapter he tells a parable about a servant who has worked all day. He has to come home and feed his master first and the master does not even thank him. Jesus says that this was right because that is what servants are supposed to do. They are unworthy people doing their duty. Even though it sounds harsh to us, he was emphasizing that forgiving is our responsibility. It is something we are supposed to do and it is not much influenced by how others respond to us. It almost seems that forgiveness is a one-way street. We are responsible to forgive, whatever is done to us and however the person responds after.

This means that in spite of the brief and rather unsatisfactory exchange in the parking lot, the responsibility for forgiveness lies with Bert. It is his Christian duty to do what he can to be at peace with Salvatore. It is quite likely he may need more in-depth interaction to bring full resolution, but he can work at not holding this against him and seek to overcome the evil with good. In the process, he needs to work towards the goal of understanding Salvatore, learning to value him, and loving him genuinely. By the same token, Salvatore needs to go through a genuine experience of conviction so he can deal with the repentance and forgiveness problem with Bert.

Does this mean that Bert should forgive and forget? That is what Salvatore requested, but does this make sense? In Jeremiah 31:34 God says that he will forgive our wickedness and will remember our sins no more. What does "remember" mean in this verse? First, we need to note that God is eternal and infinite. He does not forget like we do. His capacities are such that nothing escapes his mind or his memory. So when he talks about not remembering our sins, he is not referring to memory. Obviously, God knows what we have done and where we have fallen short. Whether it was yesterday, last week, or last year, it is not out of his memory. But when we are Christians, he does not hold our sin against us. It is not over our head or staring us in the face. His forgiveness keeps our slate clean. From a human perspective, the issues are somewhat similar. If we have a brain and a memory, past events will still be retained but the question is whether we hold them against others.

Philippians 3:13, where Paul talks about forgetting what is behind, is often cited to support the "forgive and forget" theory. It is interesting to note that early in the same chapter Paul talks about his background, how he was circumcised, of the people of Israel, of the tribe of Benjamin, a Hebrew, a Pharisee, along with a number of other historical facts. Then he talks about taking all these historical issues and weighing them up against the knowledge of Christ. He uses the image of profit and loss to discuss this. His history comes out as loss and Christ comes out as profit. In that context, he says that he is forgetting the past. Again, he is not wiping his past from his memory. In fact, if he had obliterated it from memory he would not have been able to talk about it early in the chapter. He is not counting it as crucial. It is not running his life. He is not going to rely on his past successes.

Passive, Aggressive, and Assertive Responses

One of the dangers in a book like this is that the reader could get the impression that you cannot confront anyone about anything. If you are upset with someone, you should simply keep it to yourself and deal with your own goals, expectations, and so on. But this is not the right approach. The key is that we need to approach others in a way that is consistent with a commitment to righteousness. What we need to do is look at three different communication styles—passive, aggressive, and assertive.

The passive or nonassertive approach to communication focuses on seeking to please others by yielding, placating, or giving in. People who adopt this approach to relationships will tend to implode their anger because they do not want to run the risk of losing the relationship. This would result in the blocking of their needs to be accepted, appreciated, and affirmed. They tend to bury their vengeance and to inaccurately think they have forgiven the other person, even though the anger is still raging inside.

The aggressive approach to communication looks exactly the opposite. The emphasis is on getting your own way and making demands on others. People who adopt this approach will tend to explode with their anger and become quite overbearing toward others. They tend not to respect others or value them and their major relational style is control and dominance. Often they will have others who will get along with them, but only because the aggressive people have exerted their power.

It is not uncommon for people to fluctuate between passivity and aggressiveness. I remember dealing with an associate pastor a number of years ago who would let things accumulate over time and appear to be quite tolerant. Then all of a sudden, or so it seemed, he would lash out at people and become quite overbearing. In the community he created an atmosphere of unpredictability because people were not sure which side they were going to see. At one moment his anger seemed under control, and at the next it was raging.

The third style is the assertive one. In a sense, this is a compromise position between the two extremes. The emphasis is on respect for one's own values and convictions along with those held by others. Power is shared so that one person or opinion does not dominate or become subservient. When assertive people become angry they do not lash out and blame others. Nor do they internalize what they are feeling and never bring it out into the open. They are willing to experience the risk in community by sharing what they are going through with integrity.

Clearly, Salvatore adopted the aggressive style and exploded his anger on to Bert. Control and dominance were such that Bert was not even able to express himself or offer a counterargument. Salvatore could have adopted the passive approach and just gone into a quiet burn. This might have covered the vengeance behaviorally, but he would probably have experienced it in attitude. The ideal, of course, would have been the assertive approach. He could have invited Bert out for coffee, asked him his perspective on the class, and given some of his own opinions. This style would have allowed him to express his own opinions, but it would have afforded Bert the opportunity to express his.

In sum, these concepts revolve around three words—freedom, worth, and community. In a healthy relationship there is a permission for freedom. Each person is free to experience and express their experiences. There is also a communication of worth. When freedom is exercised, both the person who is expressing their experience and the person who is the recipient communicate a sense of value and worth, both of themselves and each other. Finally, there is an affirmation of community. Both parties act and react in a way that facilitates the relationship so that neither person is negated or disaffirmed. When we express our anger in this kind of a context, it becomes more of a facilitator than an inhibitor.

Personal Reflections

1. The "sharing concerns" syndrome is rampant in many evangelical churches. Do you find yourself "sharing concerns" in a hostile way? Is there a more accurate way to describe what you are doing? Have you ever been on the receiving end of this? What did it feel like?
2. The next time you confront someone or are confronted by someone, separate the content from the style. Often problems are created because of the way we confront, not because of the content. As you reflect on the Bert–Salvatore interaction, list a number of stylistic alternatives that could have been utilized to make this a more productive exchange for both parties.
3. Commit the words of Romans 12:17–21 to memory. This is a wonderful passage to bring to communal life and the messiness of relationships.
4. List some relationships where you have tried everything to bring resolution and found that you were unsuccessful. What feelings does that produce in you? Do you feel regret? remorse? guilt? discomfort? a lack of resolution? How do the words of Romans 12:18 impact these situations?
5. The biblical notion of love is behaviorally oriented. Our contemporary culture has moved love into the realm of the emotive. Reflect on this difference and write down the practical implications of this. For example, for those of us who are married, loving your

spouse will be understood in very different ways, depending on the definition we bring to the word "love."
6. Take a concordance or word study book and trace the teaching about forgiveness in the Bible. Focus on both the vertical and horizontal components of it. List some of the specific behaviors that forgiveness requires and demands. How might these show themselves in your everyday life?
7. Luke 17 puts the responsibility for forgiveness with the offended rather than with the offender. In some sense this flies in the face of our sense of justice. Think of a relationship where you have really had to work at forgiveness. Has the other person responded in ways that you have found facilitating? Have you felt a lack of response from them? How can the words of Luke 17 inform this relationship so you both experience more freedom?
8. Because of some inaccurate teaching on anger, some Christians believe that the passive communication style is the best one. Why do you think this might be? Is there any part of biblical theology that would lead us to be negating what we believe and think?
9. Do you know any aggressive people? What does it feel like to be on the receiving end of their bulldozing? What do you feel about yourself when they act this way? Can you level with any of them and let them know how you feel?
10. We have suggested that assertiveness affirms freedom, worth, and community. List some of the qualities or characteristics involved in assertive responses. Can you work on any of these as a way of expressing your anger behaviorally?

ENDNOTES

i. *Thumos* and other derivations of the word can be found twenty times in the New Testament (Matt. 2:16; Luke 4:28; Acts 12:20; 19:28; Rom. 2:8; 2 Cor. 12:20; Gal. 5:20; Eph. 4:31; Col. 3:8; Heb. 11:27; Rev. 12:12; 14:8, 10, 19; 15:1, 7; 16:1, 19; 18:3; 19:15).

ii. *Parorgismos* and other derivations of the word can be found three times in the New Testament (Rom. 10:19; Eph. 4:26; 6:4).

iii. *Orge* and other derivations of the word can be found forty-two times in the New Testament (Matt. 3:7; 5:22; 18:34; 22:7; Mark 3:5; Luke 3:7; 14:21; 15:28; 21:23; John 3:36; Rom. 1:18; 2:5, 8; 3:5; 4:15; 5:9; 9:22; 12:19; 13:4–5; Eph. 2:3; 4:26, 31; 5:6; Col. 3:6, 8; 1 Thess. 1:10; 2:16; 5:9; 1 Tim. 2:8; Titus 1:7; Heb. 3:11; 4:3; James 1:19–20; Rev. 6:16–17; 11:18; 12:17; 14:10; 16:19; 19:15).

iv. *Aganaktesis* and other derivations of the word can be found eight times in the New Testament (Matt. 20:24; 21:15; 26:8; Mark 10:14, 41; 14:4; Luke 13:14; 2 Cor. 7:11).

REFERENCES

Augsburger, D. W. *The Freedom of Forgiveness.* Chicago: Moody, 1984.
Brand, P., and P. Yancey. *Pain: The Gift Nobody Wants.* New York: HarperCollins, 1993.
Lerner, H. G. *The Dance of Anger.* New York: Harper and Row, 1985.

FURTHER READING

Augsburger, D. W. *Anger and Assertiveness in Pastoral Care*. Philadelphia: Fortress, 1979. Examines ways to channel anger with constructive communication strategies.

———. *The Freedom of Forgiveness*. Chicago: Moody, 1984. A simple book that outlines the freedom that Christians experience when they are willing to pay the price of forgiveness.

Brand, P. and P. Yancey. *Pain: The Gift Nobody Wants*. New York: HarperCollins, 1993. An excellent discussion of pain with insights transferable to emotional pain.

Carlson, D. L. *Overcoming Hurts and Anger*. Eugene, Oreg.: Harvest House, 1981. Deals broadly with negative emotions, providing some good biblical understanding and helpful ways to think about anger.

Dryden, W. *Dealing with Anger Problems*. Sarasota, Fla.: Professional Resource Exchange, 1990. Presents a rational-emotive approach to anger in the form of a guidebook that provides counselors with specific interventions.

Fein, M. L. *Integrated Anger Management*. Westport, Conn.: Praeger, 1993. Discusses the positive aspects of anger and the way to utilize it in social situations.

Hargrave, T. D. *Families and Forgiveness*. New York: Brunner/Mazel, 1994. Describes therapeutic process to move clients from insight, understanding, and compensation to forgiveness in the context of their families.

Lerner, H. G. *The Dance of Anger*. New York: Harper and Row, 1985. Although the primary focus of this book is anger and women, it is a helpful tool for understanding anger in all relationships.

Lewis, C. S. *God in the Dock: Essays on Theology and Ethics*. Grand Rapids: Eerdmans, 1970. Contains one of Lewis's famous essays on the modern approach to God that puts humanity in the role of judge and God in the courtroom dock.

Oliver, G. J., and H. N. Wright, *When Anger Hits Home*. Chicago: Moody, 1992. A helpful discussion of anger in the family and of the myths and the gift of anger.

Potter-Efron, R. and P. *Letting Go of Anger*. Oakland: New Harbinger, 1995. Focuses on styles of anger by providing readers with self-tests.

Further Reading

Rainey, S. B. *Anger.* Colorado Springs: NavPress, 1992. Discussion guide style of book that approaches anger in the Institute of Biblical Counseling (Larry Crabb) framework.

Simon, S. B. and S. *Forgiveness.* New York: Warner, 1990. Practical book that teaches that forgiveness is a sign of emotional strength and is the antidote to making peace with our past.

Smedes, L. B. *Forgive and Forget.* New York: Harper and Row, 1984. Guides the reader through four major steps toward forgiveness—hurting, hating, healing, and reconciliation.

Stoop, D., and S. Arterburn, *The Angry Man.* Vancouver: Word, 1991. This book helps us to see the origins of anger and to move toward healing in new ways to relate.

Warren, N. C. *Make Anger Your Ally.* Colorado Springs: Focus on the Family, 1990. Helpful in understanding the physiology of anger with many illustrations that help one to visualize success in dealing with anger.

LaVergne, TN USA
10 March 2011
219645LV00001B/12/A